Rage & Reconciliation

Medical Humanities

Thomas Mayo, series editor

Rage & Reconciliation

Inspiring a Health Care Revolution

Edited by
LEE GUTKIND

SOUTHERN METHODIST
UNIVERSITY PRESS
Dallas

Requests for permission to reproduce material from this work should be sent to:

Rights and Permissions

Southern Methodist University Press

PO Box 750415

Dallas, Texas 75275-0415

Cover and text design by Tom Dawson

Library of Congress Cataloging-in-Publication Data

Rage and reconciliation : inspiring a health care revolution / edited by Lee Gutkind.

p. cm.— (Medical humanities series)

ISBN 0-87074-503-4 (pbk. : alk. paper)

1. Medical errors. 2. Medical errors—Anecdotes. 3. Medical care—Quality control—Anecdotes. 4. Medical ethics. I. Gutkind, Lee. II Series.

R729.8.R34 2005

610—dc22   2005051579

Printed in the United States of America on acid-free paper

10 9 8 7 6 5 4 3 2 1

Contents

Editor's Note

In 2002, the Jewish Healthcare Foundation offered a $10,000 writer's prize for the best original essay for a special issue of *Creative Nonfiction* to focus on patients' rights and medical mishaps. The call for manuscripts resulted in over four hundred submissions—a testament to the prize, of course, but also to the topic. As it turned out, writers on all sides of the issue, including doctors, patients, lawyers, and even HMO administrators, had much to say about the state of patient care.

The prize went to attorney Ruthann Robson's entry, "Notes from a Difficult Case," and in 2003, that story and ten other intense and moving personal essays were published as issue #21 of *Creative Nonfiction*, entitled *Rage and Reconciliation: Inspiring a Health Care Revolution.*

This new book includes all of the essays originally published in the journal, with the addition of five new essays and a CD containing professional readings of three of the works and a panel discussion of the ethical issues raised by the essays.

A foreword by Karen Wolk Feinstein, President of the Jewish Healthcare Foundation and Chair of the Pittsburgh Regional Healthcare Initiative, explains the original goals behind the project—goals that the journal fulfilled and that, we hope, the publication of this new book will continue. We hope that the transformation of *Rage and Reconciliation* into this more permanent format will attract an even greater audience for this important and timely topic and will make a significant contribution toward reducing medical errors and putting patients' needs first.

L.G., 2005

Close Encounters of the Worst Kind

An Intimate Look at Medical Error

Karen Wolk Feinstein

∽

You may ask: Why would a health foundation commission an issue of a literary journal meant to focus on medical mishaps and system failures — and sponsor a $10,000 prize for one of the essays?

Such a publication would be sad reading, to be sure. After all, haven't we all seen the statistics? An estimated 100,000 people die every year from preventable medical errors. More are seriously injured, some permanently.

In 2002, when the Jewish Healthcare Foundation decided to sponsor a writer's prize for a special issue of *Creative Nonfiction,* we hoped to help people hear the stories and picture the faces behind the statistics and sense the tragedy of these losses. We wanted readers to experience medical errors from both the patient and the physician perspectives. We wanted to bring to light the emotional and physical costs of weak doctor-patient relationships, whatever the cause (and the causes are often multiple). We expected that the essays would raise tough questions: Couldn't we work together to ensure that these things don't happen again? Would we acknowledge our imperative to fix things that are broken—appropriately and with consideration for all parties involved?

Such a fix, of course, would require an institutional will to deliver perfect patient care and overcome current inertia and denial. We can prevent many of the errors and bad practices that cause the human suffering the stories explore, but any solution will require our support of professionals and organizations that take on this challenge.

FOREWORD

In the Pittsburgh region, the Jewish Healthcare Foundation does many things to advance good work design proven to eradicate medical errors and wasteful and harmful practices, putting the patient first. The Pittsburgh Regional Healthcare Initiative builds safe environments for physicians and health professionals to report errors, trace each to its root cause, test and implement solutions, and share lessons from each experience.

Enormous benefits accrue when teams in highly complex environments have the will to do what is right with precision. Consider the aviation industry, which makes it simple for a pilot to report an error—and in fact penalizes the pilot who fails to do so. Process improvement in health care will reap tremendous benefits. For example, the American Society of Anesthesiologists has supported a massive redesign of its work in response to a rising litigation crisis; doctors now work in teams, monitoring themselves and structuring their own solutions to approach error-free practice.

This issue of *Creative Nonfiction*—now this book—will, we hope, give both patients and health professionals an intimate understanding of the tragedy of suboptimal practice, the futility of preventing errors through litigation, the need for protections that encourage error reporting and rapid problem solving, and the resolute leadership required among practitioners.

We should gain determination from mishaps such as those recounted here. We can and must support those who engage in diligent practice that puts patients' interests first.

•

Karen Wolk Feinstein, PhD, is President of the Jewish Healthcare Foundation and Chair of the Pittsburgh Regional Healthcare Initiative

Introduction

The Rage That Inspires Reconciliation

Lee Gutkind

∾

From 1985 through 1989, while writing a book about the organ transplant world, I watched, close-up, at arm's reach, many dozens of organ transplants: kidney, heart, liver, heart-lung and heart-liver transplants. These procedures usually took place in the middle of the night at Presbyterian-University Hospital in Pittsburgh, today part of UPMC (University of Pittsburgh Medical Center), then and perhaps now the largest organ transplant center in the world.

The scene for almost all of these procedures was very dramatic, just like in the movies. The helicopter landed on the roof of the building, usually at the point when the recipient's diseased organ had been removed—a process that had consumed perhaps four hours of cutting and suction and blood and focused concentration by three or sometimes four intense surgeons, masked and cloaked in hospital blue. A few minutes later, the rear door of the OR would fly open and the organ transplant coordinator, who had traveled from a hospital hundreds or even thousands of miles from Pittsburgh, rushed into the OR, he too masked and cloaked in blue, and deposited a small red-and-white Igloo cooler on a stainless steel table.

Then the surgeons who had removed the diseased organ from the dying candidate in Pittsburgh opened the lid of the cooler, lifted the organ with both hands and carried it to another stainless steel table to be cleaned and examined. In a few minutes, that organ, the organ from a brain-dead human being who would never walk, talk, speak or think again, who no more than six or eight hours before had been an otherwise healthy person, would be placed inside the body of the recipient. At this particular point in the procedure, I was, invariably, awestruck, even though I had witnessed many of these procedures in Pittsburgh and elsewhere in the U.S. and abroad. Three powerful images return to me when I think back more than a dozen years to those moments:

First, the removal of the diseased organ from the candidate. It isn't the removal itself that pierces my memory so much as the gaping hole it leaves behind in the patient. Picture a human being, a person you have spent hours or weeks (or years, in some cases) talking with, now lying partially naked on a stainless steel table, chest cracked and pulled apart. Look down into the bloody, bubbling cavern where the heart and/or the lungs had once sustained life. The experience is both bizarre and breathtaking. (A liver removal is less dramatic, but often more bloody.)

At this moment, the person . . . is not really a person. This person, man or woman, adult or child, is in artificial life support limbo. If something goes wrong, the old organ or organs cannot easily be returned to the body, and even if they could be, they are so decimated by disease that they would, in a matter of days or hours—or minutes—kill the patient. The new organ must work, or the patient will die. (The patient may die even if the new organ works, but that's another story.)

Then comes the placing of the new organs. That's the second powerful image I retain: the moment when the heart or heart-lung or liver is lifted out of the Igloo cooler, carried across the room and put into that dramatic gaping hole, that hole your eyes have locked onto, the hole which symbolizes a crossroads in the candidate's existence.

That carrying across the room part always made me hold my breath and triggered outlandish fantasies. What would happen if the surgeon dropped the organ, tripping and falling, like in a Three Stooges movie, the heart or liver flying up into the air and bouncing against the ceiling? The irony overwhelmed me: all of this advanced technology, an amazing cutting-edge procedure, but the surgeons, those men and women with the golden hands, could slip or fall or become distracted or become overly excited—and crush the precious, fragile organ in their bare hands! I never saw it happen or heard of it happening, but it was possible, wasn't it? We are all human and we all make mistakes. Even surgeons.

Now finally the new organ is inside the body and the surgeons begin the arduous procedure—anywhere from four to twelve hours of sewing and cutting and cauterizing, fighting sudden geysers of blood and a frightening array of other possible hazards. I witnessed a few catastrophes in the operating room: patients dying, surgeons, their hospital blues soaked in red, desperate and heroic in their fight and then dejected and decimated when they realized beyond a doubt that their fight was over and they were failing. Even at their best and brightest moments, surgeons cannot achieve the impossible.

But mostly, at this point—especially as procedures became more refined over the years I spent immersed in the world of organ transplantation—the suspense and the arduous hours in the OR led to triumph and a satisfying, exhilarating culmination. The most vivid moment of all, the moment that remains most powerfully in my mind, occurred during heart or heart-lung transplants, when, after being reattached, the new organ or organs would come back to life.

Once I witnessed a long heart-lung procedure during which, after the organs had been reconnected and the recipient's blood was finally circulating in the heart and lungs of the donor, there was a long moment when nothing happened. Total stillness and silence and waiting. I recall this moment in slow motion, as the masked and anonymous surgeon, gowned like a priest, reached across the table, placed his gloved hand into his patient's chest and casually tweaked the transplanted heart with his forefinger and thumb—an almost cavalier gesture—and immediately, amazingly, the frozen heart was set in motion and began to beat. And then the lungs began to fill with air—and move, *breathe*—at first sluggishly, and then, still as if in slow motion, they expanded and contracted more vigorously until you could hear them popping with every succeeding breath.

I remember what one of the early organ transplant surgeon pioneers, Keith Reemstma, of Columbia Presbyterian University Hospital, used to say at this point, after completing a transplant and waiting for the heart to awaken. He was a tall, gaunt, gray-haired gentleman, resembling a bank president, very unlike the average transplant surgeon. Reemstma would clear his throat and shake his head and then pause for effect with a certain amount of arrogance and pride, before announcing: "Well, it's just another goddamn miracle."

For many transplant recipients, however, the miracle ended at that point. Even in the most perfect scenarios, recipients invariably lived through weeks or months and sometimes years of difficult, painful, depressing rehabilitation necessitating repeated readmissions to the hospital and sometimes dozens of additional procedures, including retransplant. There were, and still are, liver transplant recipients who had to endure four or even five retransplants.

Although immunosuppressive medications (antirejection drugs) are becoming increasingly effective, they are not without their own evils. While fighting rejection, they can at the same time precipitate devastating consequences. Among other things, antirejection drugs can cause crippling osteoporosis or life-threatening diseases such as lymphoma. They can also devastate a kidney or the pancreas, leading to the doom and gloom of further organ transplants for the patient.

After the miracle, the potential for failure haunts the recipient's every waking moment. The survival rates that surgeons usually mentioned when being interviewed by reporters at the time—perhaps 80 percent or even 90 percent—sounded terrific, justifying the potential complications from the difficult procedures. But those cheery-sounding numbers were one-year survival rates: one year after the organ was transplanted. Even today, although the records are somewhat incomplete, ten-year survival rates for heart and liver transplantation hover at only around the 50 percent mark. The miracle remains vivid for half of those recipients; for the other unlucky half, the miracle dissipates and dies.

For my book *Many Sleepless Nights: The World of Organ Transplantation* I followed approximately twenty candidates and recipients from the moment they arrived in Pittsburgh to be evaluated as candidates until the transplant procedure was complete. A few of them died waiting for an organ, and by the time the book was published in 1989 and then republished again in paperback in 1991, more than half of the patients I had followed were dead. Today, as far as I can tell, no more than three of the recipients about whom I wrote in any detail are still breathing.

I was not deterred by the demise of the people I wrote about during those transplant years. On the contrary, I was intrigued enough by the medical world to write three more books about it over the next seven years. By and large, the surgeons I spent time with profoundly influenced my choice of subjects for two of those books—albeit in a rather negative way. I noticed, for example, that some transplant surgeons, more often the liver guys, were much less interested in pediatric patients than they were adult patients.

The liver transplant team usually rounded in the late afternoons. We always met on the seventh floor of Presby, which was the main liver transplant unit, and then worked our way up or down from there. This was in the early days of transplantation, so in addition to the Pittsburgh team, there were surgeons who had come to Pittsburgh from all over the world to see if and how organ transplantation and antirejection medications worked. Sometimes forty or more surgeons would round in a pack, a white-coated army marching into the transplant wards. The patients and families waiting to see their doctors in the late afternoon—some of whom had been waiting for hours—referred to this group as the "Thundering Horde."

The last stop on rounds was on the second floor in the Intensive Care Unit (ICU). Here lay the most devastated of the patients, plugged into monitors and hoses, on the edge of death. At the far end of the ICU there was an aboveground tunnel that led from Presby to Children's Hospital. This was the Bahnson Bridge, named for Presby's longtime chief of surgery, Henry Bahnson, who, as legend had it, had insisted that the bridge be built so that he and his staff, when rounding, needn't walk outside, down and up a flight of stairs in the middle of those bitter Pittsburgh winters with nothing but their white lab coats or scrubs to protect them. Those were the days when surgeons could demand and receive extravagances—even bridges—at the blink of an eye. But Bahnson had an ulterior motive. He was hoping that more surgeons would find it easier to walk across that bridge and care for the kids and not have an excuse for avoiding the pediatric patients. As it turned out, convenience wasn't the issue; when the "attending" leading rounds departed the ICU and headed toward the Bahnson Bridge, at least two-thirds of the Thundering Horde would turn around and walk the other way.

I once asked one of those disappearing surgeons why he and so many of his colleagues avoided the Bahnson Bridge when the liver transplant team still had pediatric cases to see. This was a surgeon who had helped me to understand some of the more complicated surgical procedures I had witnessed in the OR over the past few months. But he didn't seem inclined to help me to understand his disinterest in crossing the Bahnson Bridge. "Because," he said simply, "they are children." I looked at him quizzically and nodded. "Children," he said, shaking his head dismissively and looking right back at me, "are different." This man was not being perverse or arrogant, I was to find out. He was stating a fact.

This was enough to propel me across the Bahnson Bridge on my own and into the world of Children's Hospital—and to plunge me into another book. After my transplant immersion experience was finished and *Many Sleepless Nights* was published, I immersed myself for two additional years in a high-acuity pediatric facility to find out what exactly this surgeon was talking about—why children, human beings with arms and legs and heads and eyes, miniatures of adults, were so different.

While researching *One Children's Place,* I discovered that children were, in fact, very different than adult patients, mostly in obvious ways. They were smaller and much more fragile, requiring more meticulous and gentle treatment both in and out of surgery. Children weren't, as I had so quickly assumed, miniatures of adults. The problems and challenges of care and treatment, not just in surgery but also throughout the realm of medicine, were considerably different. Children were also often better patients. Adults were sometimes vulgar and nasty. Children, for the most part, were polite. When they were annoyed or in pain, they rarely complained; mostly, they cried— and broke your heart.

I strongly suspect that that's the other reason that many of the surgeons did not cross the Bahnson Bridge: They were protecting their hearts. It was difficult enough to see patients suffer or die, to become significantly attached and then to lose them and, justifiably or not, to feel somewhat responsible for that loss. But losing children who are patients, especially if you yourself were a parent, as were many of these surgeons, was, perhaps, too much to take. Especially in organ transplantation, where two of ten of your patients are gone every year despite your best efforts, and half of your patients have expired within a decade.

"Yes," a surgeon can say, "I gave them those ten years. Without me, or someone like me, maybe they wouldn't have grown up, studied Shakespeare, watched the Red Sox win the World Series and graduated from high school at the head of their class. Maybe they wouldn't have experienced sexual pleasure—the ups and downs of marriage—and even the joys of having their own children to bond with." This is imperative solace for surgeons sometimes. But it's subtle.

There's another image from my transplant years that I can't seem to purge from my mind—a scenario that was invariably repeated in the transplant wards during rounds in the days, weeks and sometimes months after the "miracle" in the OR. When the Thundering Horde came into a patient's room, they often turned their backs on the patient and clustered around a complicated wall chart, studying numbers gathered by nurses and residents that showed the way the body was responding to the immunosuppressive medications. Conversations about "the numbers" and whether the doses of medication should be adjusted might go on for ten minutes or more. From time to time, the transplant team answered questions posed by the visiting surgeons. Decisions about adjusting medications were made and noted on the chart. Then the Thundering Horde would turn abruptly and march down the hall to the next room, often without a word to the patient or the concerned family members.

Once, I heard an attending surgeon reprimand a resident for talking too long with a patient when there were so many others to see. "Save lives first, answer questions later," he said.

To be fair, the patients and families acknowledged the truth in that statement. The surgeons were so busy jetting through the night to retrieve organs, then standing on their feet in the operating room to implant them, then rounding to make certain their patients' immunosuppressive medications were effective, that they couldn't really afford to invest time or energy in actual, friendly conversation, even if that give-and-take might have made the patients feel better and their loved ones feel more secure. Still, understanding why the transplant team members were often so rude and insensitive did not eradicate the hurt and resentment the behavior caused. I remember one patient commenting with great bitterness, "My doctors know what my liver looks like, but not my face."

The surgeons' reluctance to interact sympathetically with patients and families did not stop at the Bahnson Bridge. During my two years at Children's Hospital, I witnessed many surgeons locking horns with angry and dissatisfied parents, mostly mothers, who didn't feel they were getting enough information to understand what was happening to their children. Surgeons were also frequently in combat with house pediatricians who constantly urged their colleagues to be more tactful and less aggressive with families of chronically ill children.

The chief of surgery at Children's at the time I was in residence—I'll call him Leonard Levine—readily acknowledged the importance of sensitivity while debating its practicality. He had a very tender, compassionate side, which he often held under lock and key. "Sometimes I get very attached to parents [of my patients]. Sometimes I feel as close to them as I do my own family," he told me. "But I won't let that sway me. I will dump on them in a minute because basically I am cold-blooded as hell about one thing. I am trying to get their kid to live. . . . Psychological trauma and all that stuff is important, but it doesn't made a goddamn bit of difference if you are well adjusted—and dead."

It was that comment and a few more like it that eventually led me to my third book written from the inside of the health-care system. For this book, *Stuck in Time: The Tragedy of Childhood Mental Illness*, I immersed myself in a psychiatric institution for another two years to write about children with severe mental health problems—and their families. During that period in the middle 1990s, I learned, among many other things, how wrong Leonard Levine had been in his scale of values in relation to emotional stability. The patients I spent time with were, primarily, hard-core cases—with bipolar, borderline personality and schizophrenic diagnoses. Most of these children were perfectly fit and healthy physical specimens, debilitated only by the ravages of their medications. But nearly every one of them—depressed, confused and desperate—would have chosen, and frequently did choose, death (or attempts at death) over the emotional trauma of being alive. I understand that their self-mutilation and attempts at suicide were part of their illness, but it takes a particularly insensitive brand of arrogance to insist that emotional health is less critical than physical well-being. We all know now that the body and the mind are in constant and inevitable synchronization.

But the world is considerably more complicated now, in 2005, than it was a decade ago. Health-care costs are out of control, and competition for the available health-care dollar is heated. "Surgeon" and "doctor" are no longer the elitist and all-powerful words they once were, and these esteemed individuals are no longer immune from criticism and blame. The essays in this collection reflect this new, honest and refreshing reality. Natalie Smith Parra and Cornelia Reynolds fight wars against physicians' arrogance and a reluctant and inflexible system. Ruthann Robson, in "Notes from a Difficult Case," refuses to be stonewalled, ridiculed or misled by her surgeons, her oncologists, her phlebotomists—and through her own sheer persistence and force of will she keeps herself alive. For an essay about her struggle, Robson was awarded a $10,000 prize, donated by the Jewish Healthcare Foundation, for the best original essay by an emerging writer.

Most of the essays in this collection were originally published in the literary journal I edit, *Creative Nonfiction,* in its twenty-first issue, entitled *Rage and Reconciliation: Inspiring a Healthcare Debate.* Within a few months of publication, we sold out of the issue. Then I approached the editors of Southern Methodist University Press to consider publishing the collection as a book. SMU Press was starting a medical humanities series edited by Tom Mayo, a professor in the SMU law school, whose specialties are health law and medical ethics. The director of the Press, Keith Gregory, is himself a heart transplant recipient.

For this collection we added four new essays, beginning with "A Measure of Acceptance" by Floyd Skloot, a victim of Epstein-Barr virus, who relates the depressing and humiliating battery of tests he must endure when the government questions his disabled status—and threatens to reduce the disability payments that support him and his wife. The right of all Americans to have adequate health care is much discussed in Washington and the news; Skloot's experience suggests that we should also have the right to receive help from the government if we are truly disabled. In "Rachel at Work: A Mother's Report," Jane Bernstein examines whether we all, including the retarded, have the right to work. The ideas and issues Bernstein captures and confronts fall clearly under the broad rubric of patients' rights and the severity of the unwieldy system that restricts us.

The remaining two new essays in this collection were written by physicians: Margaret Overton, an anesthesiologist practicing in Chicago, and Helena Studer, a former pediatrician. In her vivid essay, "The Burden of Baby Boy Smith," Dr. Studer describes one of the experiences that led her to quit practicing medicine for reasons primarily related to the difficult decisions that confront physicians every day—and the lack of guidance, support and alternatives provided for doctors in the process of making those decisions. Ron Grant, another pediatrician who walked away from his profession, especially touched me with his essay, "Hypoplastic Heart," which begins with Grant driving a three-week-old baby to the morgue in his Jeep. The parents, we learn, had two viable options for their child: "a heart transplant or a natural death in the comfort of his home." They chose the latter, a decision that forced Grant, as well, to question the cost, in quality of life, of technological advances like organ transplantation.

The medical community has long avoided criticism and examination, at least to a certain extent, but now, after a century of stonewalling, it is comforting to realize that doctors themselves are beginning to acknowledge their own vulnerabilities—and their mistakes. Linda Peeno, author of "Burden of Oath," is a physician who insists that her only patient is our seriously ill health-care system. Her experience as a medical reviewer for a prominent HMO—and the loss of her position—were the subject of *Damaged Care,* a television movie starring Laura Dern. Richard Beach is a neonatologist who dares to criticize his colleagues, ignoring the threat this behavior poses to his career and livelihood. The ironies of medicine and the heartache of pain and suffering are also explored in essays by Deborah McDonald, Nancy Linnon and others. The essays collected in *Rage and Reconciliation* were not commissioned. They were submitted to us, nearly four hundred of them over the course of six months.

The kind of confession and communication that occurs in *Rage and Reconciliation* is rare—so rare that I wanted to enhance its impact by bringing these often-disparate groups together in Pittsburgh, the home of *Creative Nonfiction*. With financial help from a number of foundations, we arranged for professional actors to prepare some of the essays presented in this collection and read them aloud, dramatically, in front of a full-house audience at the City Theater. We also invited prominent members of the health-care community, including physicians, ethicists and administrators, to comment about and debate some of the issues inherent in the essays that were read, with the authors and the audience participating. It was a lively, sometimes angry and emotional discussion, and the CD included with *Rage and Reconciliation* captures it vividly for the readers of this collection.

After the readings and the dialogue that followed, I think we all experienced a special sense of satisfaction. A connection had been made among all of the parties involved; a link had been established among the patients who felt wronged, the physicians who felt misunderstood, the actors who attempted to bridge the gap between the opposing parties, and the writers who had exposed their souls to the world. At the reception after the program, we drank wine and beer and coffee and shared the exhilaration of the moment.

I remember thinking, as I sat in the corner watching the groups come together and listening to their conversations, that a slight change had taken place. Something small but significant had happened. I am not saying that the event precipitated a change. But the dialogue reflected clarity and a sanity that superseded the perception of the physicians' arrogance and the helplessness patients felt in the past. The fact that we, a tiny journal, were able to influence a large and powerful health-care organization (the Jewish Health-care Foundation) to contribute support for a literary endeavor, the fact that we received four hundred very intense essays linking patients, nurses, social workers and doctors, the fact that in these essays doctors were willing to express frustration, anger and vulnerability—all of this indicated that a new attitude was emerging, an attitude captured by this dramatic moment. The rage of the past is dissipating slowly and being replaced by an essential awareness that reconciliation is inevitable and vital if the health-care heartache in America is to be confronted and controlled.

Notes from a Difficult Case

Ruthann Robson

∾

Almost everyone I know advised me to sue. Their advice was not casual, because almost everyone I know is an attorney. As am I.

At forty-two, I'd been an attorney almost half my life.

At forty-two, the doctors let it be known that I was far advanced into what would be the second half of my abbreviated life.

These were not just any doctors; these were the doctors at a world famous cancer center.

If I'd been charged with a heinous crime, I would have retained the best criminal defense attorney I could find. Convicted of a rare cancer, I sought the best advocates for my appeal.

The doctors at the famous cancer center pronounced mine a difficult case.

My tumor was inoperable, the cancer had metastasized to my liver, and the only possible treatment was a highly toxic regimen of chemotherapy. If the chemotherapy infusions were not successful, I had no chance of survival.

The doctors at the world famous cancer center were correct in their prediction regarding the chemotherapy: it failed to shrink the twenty-pound tumor that distended my abdomen even more pronouncedly now that I had lost thirty pounds after four cycles of chemotherapy.

But they were incorrect about almost everything else.

My tumor was not inoperable.

My cancer had not metastasized to my liver.

Chemotherapy had never been successful on a cancer such as mine.

I turned forty-three. Forty-four. Forty-five.

The circumstances of my ordeal are both simple and complicated. They could be allegations on a complaint, numbered and neat, and augmented by specific dates and quotes from the defendants' own records:

1. On such and such a date, the patient plaintiff was seen by the Chief Sarcoma Surgeon, who observed that the plaintiff had a "very large abdominal mass and lesions in the liver consistent with liver metastases."

2. On a date approximately a week later, the patient underwent a liver biopsy, for which the cytology report read "suspicious cells present" on "*scanty* evidence" (emphasis added).

3. On a date approximately another week later, the patient plaintiff was seen by the oncologist, who told her that she had an "extensive intra-abdominal, presumed soft tissue sarcoma, probable liposarcoma, with hepatic metastases" with no "curative potential," and "no role for surgical intervention at this time, given the presence of metastatic disease."

4. On yet another date yet another week later, the patient was ordered to have a biopsy of the *abdominal mass*, the surgical pathology report for which was *liver biopsy* with the diagnosis of "well-differentiated lipoma-like sarcoma."

Meaning that within these four weeks, the patient was first diagnosed with liver metastases by the famous sarcoma surgeon, given a liver biopsy to confirm this judgment on "scanty evidence" that showed "suspicious cells," then told she was incurable by the oncologist because of liver metastases, and then given another biopsy of the abdominal tumor, which was mislabeled a biopsy of the liver.

In other words, the doctors screwed up their biopsies.

Later, the complaint would introduce the expert opinions from oncologists and oncology textbooks.

32. There has never been a case in which liposarcoma has metastasized to the liver.

33. Well-differentiated liposarcoma is a nonmetastasizing lesion.

34. Chemotherapy is ineffective on well-differentiated liposarcoma.

In other words, the doctors screwed up more than the biopsies.

The doctors at the famous cancer center were wrong when they pronounced me hopeless, incurable, and inoperable because of liver metastases, not knowing that liposarcoma, in its well-differentiated state, does not metastasize. Even if it becomes poorly differentiated, liposarcoma does not metastasize to the liver. I was misdiagnosed and mistreated.

"Screwing up," translated into legal language, is a breach of the duty of care. "Deviation from the applicable standard of care" is one of the elements necessary to establish a cause of action for medical malpractice.

My complaint would omit facts that are not legally relevant: details that do not establish breach of the duty of care and that may not be objective or provable. I do not recall the dates of these occurrences and if they appear at all in the medical records, those narratives would differ from mine. These are the legally irrelevant facts that subsume my complaint:

• The surgeon's secretary called me and told me the liver biopsy confirmed metastasis. His secretary. Who could not answer my questions. Who did not have a soothing voice. Who was not a surgeon.

• The oncologist, when questioned, repeatedly told me that of course she/they were correct that surgery was useless because she/they were at the world famous cancer center. Though she admitted I could, perhaps, find "someone off the street to do surgery."

• The oncologist smirked—I swear—when I lost my previously waist-length hair.

• Despite my protests, I was repeatedly advised to take tranquilizers, given prescriptions for Ativan, and referred to a psychiatrist to help me deal with "it."

• A phlebotomist who stuck my emaciated arm with the needle too sharply, jabbing after he couldn't find a vein, told me I was being difficult and that I wasn't really hurt.

• I had to carry the order for the CT scan to the technicians, an order on which my doctor wrote the diagnosis "huge abdominal tumor." "Huge" was underlined. Twice.

• When I asked about the long-term effects of the chemotherapeutic agents with which I was being treated, my oncologist replied that "long-term effects" were really not the issue, and I swear it again—she smirked.

According to several studies, the decision whether or not to sue for medical malpractice is not necessarily related to the degree of the doctors' negligence or fault, or to the degree of the patient's injuries, including death.

Instead, the most consistent variable is something that is named as compassion, caring, or communication.

According to some of these same studies, only one person in thirty-five who suffers what the medical profession calls an "adverse event" decides to sue for medical malpractice.

I did not want to be the kind of person who sued.

By this I did not mean greedy, avaricious, money-hungry, gold-digging, grasping, or craven. I had become an attorney to work for the poor, turning down offers from large law firms which included bonuses of more money than I'd ever made in my life and yearly salaries that seemed to me obscene. Then I became a law professor, certainly not one of the most lucrative positions.

By this I did not mean vengeful, spiteful, savage, malicious. I knew I had the best revenge against their misdiagnosis: I had defied them and I was living and well.

By this I did not mean litigious. I admired people who sued, people who had the courage of their convictions, people who used the courts for social reform.

By this I meant damaged.

Damages are the key element in any cause for medical malpractice. It is not enough that the doctors have made mistakes; these mistakes must cause damages to the patient.

Although in some cases causation can be difficult to prove, in my difficult case, causation is unquestionable.

Damages are my difficulty.

In the medical records, the doctors note that "the patient understands that her disease is incurable."

But I did not understand. I railed and sobbed and protested. I did not sleep and could not eat, even before I succumbed to chemotherapy. I was too young and too otherwise healthy to die, wasn't I?

I lived with my imminent death for months and months. Dark days and darker nights. There were no sunsets and no sunrises during all that time. I read books I can't recall. I cursed my career, devoted to constitutional law rather than molecular biology.

Simple phrases—"planning for retirement," "after my son graduates high school," "next summer"—constricted my throat.

Trivial possessions—my hair barrette from Australia, my fountain pen with the lifetime guarantee, my *Healthy Living Cookbook*—flooded my eyes.

Pain and suffering are incalculable.

In the medical records, the doctors note that "possible chemotherapeutic options were outlined in detail. Toxicities from the chemotherapeutic agent doxorubicin/adriamycin include, but are not limited to myelosuppression and the risk of infection, mucositis, diarrhea, nausea/vomiting, and hair thinning; and from the agent ifosfamide, hemorrhagic cystitis, renal failure, and neuro-toxicity."

But they told me this was my only chance. A slim one, but the only one.

I suffered all the short-term side effects.

I weighed less than one hundred pounds and was so thin it hurt to sit on a chair. I had fevers that clawed at my bones. I was so weak I crawled down the hallway to the bathroom. I lost all my hair, even those sweet little hairs on my toes.

It's become mundane to lose one's hair.

Wear a scarf, tied jauntily. And tightly, so it doesn't slip off the slick skin.

Buy a wig; match your own color as closely as possible.

Or brave it bald and beautiful.

Don't admit to vanity.

But how to explain?

That I'd had hair to my waist for my entire life.

That the first time in my life I went to a hair salon was to get a short cut so that losing my hair would be less painful.

That it was part of my identity: "You'll recognize me at the airport. I have very long hair."

That when I was five years old, I swore I'd never cut my hair. And I didn't. Except for my annual spring split-end trim.

That I still dream of myself with long hair.

That when I see someone with hair as long as mine once was, I have to turn away.

There are long-term effects from the chemotherapy I should not have been given.

Adriamycin, an agent that is amongst chemotherapy's most toxic drugs, damages the heart muscle. My recent CT scans have revealed a new "pericardial effusion," liquid in the cavity around my heart. My regular blood tests proclaim severe and persistent anemia. My heart leaks its thinned blood as I battle to regain my balance.

Ifosfamide causes neurotoxicity. Nerve damage. I have peripheral neuropathy that is so severe some days I cannot hold a pen or strike the correct key on the keyboard. My feet, to phrase it genteelly, tingle. Not so politely, I often crumple when I try to stand, hobble when I try to walk.

Excerpts from the transcript in my possible lawsuit for wrongful chemotherapy:

Q: And what was your experience after being administered the chemotherapeutic agent adriamycin, also known as doxorubicin?

A: Also known as the "red devil." My long hair began to fall out—not "thin"—and this was accompanied by a sensation of burning on my skin, my scalp and everywhere else I had hair, as if I was being scorched with an iron set for cotton. It also produced an intense and sudden menopause with hot flashes that lasted for hours and combined with fever to make me feel as if I was on fire. I had to force myself to eat since everything tasted like the chemotherapy, which seemed to pool in my mouth even though it was administered intravenously. Nausea does not adequately describe the urge to vomit and then the vomiting. I felt as if I was being poisoned. Which I was.

Q: And what was your experience after being administered the chemotherapeutic agent ifosfamide?

A: There were many physical symptoms, nausea and intense constipation, but what was most difficult to bear was the loss of mental acuity. There seemed to be a great distance between my self and the outer world. Perhaps this is always true, but usually that distance is populated with the effluvia of daily life: a list of things to do, snatches of conversation, the last book I'd read, something I wanted to remember to say to a student or friend. But these things had evaporated, leaving a desert of immense vistas between me and the rest of the world. I struggled to be lucid, to connect, but I was intensely isolated. Everything existed on a mesa, far away and tinged with pink. . . .

Q (interrupting): Thank you. Now, did you experience any side effects from the other drugs that were administered, drugs that were intended to curtail some of the side effects of the chemotherapeutic agents?

A: Yes. (Crying). Can we take a break?

But if anyone asks me how I am, I say I am fully recovered. After I found a surgeon to remove the large abdominal tumor, I was fine.

After I underwent the experimental procedure of cryosurgery to treat the liver metastases that did not exist, I was cured and in perfect health.

When I am dizzy, I wait a moment and put my head down, casually, as if I am looking at something. When my hands are too numb to type or write and my feet too numb to walk, I am possessed of a sudden urge to read in a warm bath.

If there is a mind-body connection, then I am determined to capitalize on it.

I feel great.

I am well.

Repeat ten times. Turn around and face the four directions.

If there is an opposite term for "malingerer," that would be me.

My damages are not only impaired by my refusal to be ill, but substantially compromised by my own actions.

The day I decided to leave the oncologists at the famous cancer center and no longer follow their advice and endure their arrogance was the day I—or more correctly, my surviving family members—diminished the claim for damages.

If I had acceded to their (mis)diagnosis and (mis)treatment, I would have died. The tumor would have become so large it would have pushed against my other organs until they were dysfunctional. I would have been strangled from the inside out.

And if it were ever discovered that the lesions on my liver were not metastases but simple hemangiomas, a condition which affects 40 percent of all women, and if those surviving me had learned of my nonmetastatic liver, there would have been a terrific multimillion-dollar suit for a wrongful death resulting from medical malpractice. Economists would have testified about the worth of my life, multiplying my projected life span by my yearly salary, with expected increases and the occasional book and honorarium.

But because I disagreed, much too late in hindsight, but still soon enough to save my life, I mitigated the damages and made my case less valuable.

As the studies have shown, the decision to sue for malpractice is not necessarily motivated by money. Whether I could get one thousand dollars or ten million dollars is not the determinative factor, although it might be for any attorney I might hire, dependent as he or she would be on the contingent fee percentage of recovery.

Financially, it would seem fair to be reimbursed the fifty thousand dollars in needless chemotherapy treatments for which I and my insurance company paid the famous cancer center.

But no amount of money can compensate me for the months I had no appetites, no fun, no joy, no hope. There is no way to pay for the looks in the eyes of those who saw me: despair in the eyes of my partner, disbelief in my adolescent child, shock in my parents, the terrible pity in my coworkers and even strangers. Nothing can buy back the taste of chemical cremation that still smolders at the back of my throat.

Some studies demonstrate that the few people who choose to sue are often motivated by the altruistic desire to prevent the same fate from befalling someone else.

To save some unknown stranger.

But what are the odds that these same facts would coalesce again?

Slim to none, I assumed.

However, I later learn that a few months *before* I first went to the famous cancer center, a man a little older than I also consulted the doctors there, and was diagnosed with liposarcoma and liver metastasis. But for some reason, he went to a different hospital and found that his liver lesions were hemangiomas.

When I wasn't crying in the examining room, I argued with my oncologist at the famous cancer center. The little notebook I now carried everywhere with my medical questions was more spotted than my liver. I'd had hepatitis as a college student, couldn't the lesions on my liver be a result of that? Especially since they weren't growing, while my abdominal tumor was?

As for symptoms, I was becoming so debilitated from the chemotherapy that I felt as if my liver as well as all my other organs were barely resisting an acute failure.

No, my oncologist insisted.

No. No. No. No. No.

There is no use in denying it: your cancer has metastasized to your liver.

Even as the contrary evidence was staring her in the face.

My face, to be precise.

My lip, to be more precise. Upper lip, left quadrant.

A hemangioma.

Something that looked to me like a blood blister had appeared after an accident a few years ago. It hadn't gone away, and then after I consulted doctors, it hadn't responded to either conventional or laser surgery. When the plastic surgeon suggested plum lipstick, I decided I'd just live with a lesion on my upper lip.

Not knowing that I was also living quite fine with the same purpling on my invisible liver.

Did the oncologist even notice my face? What else did she fail to notice?

Or did she not even know what a hemangioma was?

Should I sue? Should I not?

The statute of limitations ticks like the metronome of my adriamycin-damaged heart.

All states limit the time in which a lawsuit for medical malpractice, or almost anything else, can be brought. The time for medical malpractice suits is relatively short, often shorter than for other personal injury lawsuits because legislatures have reacted to a perceived crisis—and the powerful medical profession with effective lobbyists. Having a fewer number of lawsuits is considered a good result.

This is called tort reform.

Popular with legislators everywhere.

Limit the greedy plaintiffs and their even more avaricious lawyers; protect our innocent doctors, hospitals, and HMOs.

After a study showing that medical malpractice awards have been larger in the past few years, some legislatures place a cap on damages awards.

After a study showing that one in eight people are seriously injured during their hospitalizations by acts of medical personnel, most legislatures do nothing.

As for medical insurance, any legislative action is viewed as tantamount to communism.

My medical insurance refused to allow me to see a doctor "out of network." Even after the oncologists at the famous cancer center had dismissed me as hopeless and I had learned of another cancer center having great success with my type of cancer.

"There are forty thousand oncologists in our network. What makes you think you're so special you need to go elsewhere?" the nurse caseworker assigned to my difficult case asked me.

"I'm dying," I replied.

She suggested a hospice.

"I'll fight this," I vowed.

"You don't seem to understand you have a difficult case."

I went out of network. I went out of state. I would have gone out of this world. I filed the insurance claims and figured if the company didn't pay, I'd appeal. I'd resort to credit cards with high interest rates, figuring that if I died,

I wouldn't care, and if I lived, I'd be happy to worry about something as survivable as debt.

The doctors at the out-of-network cancer center saved my life.

The doctors at the out-of-network cancer center may think I am a difficult case, but they also seem to realize that I am a person who does not want to die. They do not smirk at me, although I am bald and my elbows are like arrows. They do not seem squeamish when faced with my little notebook of questions.

As if they have read my notebook, the first question the doctors at the out-of-network cancer center ask me is: "Why haven't you had surgery?"

I am so stunned that the only response that forms in the cage of my mind has something to do with the First Amendment cases I have taught about Jehovah's Witnesses, Christian Scientists, and faith healers refusing medical treatment. Luckily, this does not escape my mouth.

The surgeon at the out-of-network cancer center is a talented, careful, and knowledgeable specialist in sarcomas. I am certain that the surgery he performed was far better than any surgery that would have been performed by the surgeon at the famous cancer center who couldn't recognize a hemangioma on a CT scan and who had his secretary make his unpleasant phone calls.

This makes my prognosis, not to mention my life, much better.

This makes my legal case more difficult.

My out-of-network surgery and hospitalization cost less than my chemotherapy regimes had cost, less than a prolonged hospice would have cost. My insurance company denied my claims. I appealed. I lost. I appealed again. After a hearing at the World Trade Center, the company agreed to pay the expenses associated with saving my life, even though they were incurred out of network.

When the World Trade Center buildings collapsed, I was at the out-of-network cancer center having a follow-up CT scan performed.

Strapped into the massive white doughnut of a machine, I prayed the images it produced would be tumorless.

Mesmerized by the television sets in the waiting rooms, I prayed the images it transmitted were exaggerated.

The last section of the complaint is called the "prayer for relief."

If I decided to sue, my damages would be measured by an award; my injuries would be compensated with monetary relief.

Money.

I could not ask for an injunction. I could not request that the doctors go back to medical school or receive further training in cancer or compassion. Or that they be administered adriamycin or ifosfamide.

I would never receive an apology. And nothing I could prove would ever mean that the famous cancer center would be ordered to cease and desist its boastful advertisements.

One of the principles of medical malpractice is that the monetary awards will act as deterrents. The theory is that litigation which results in compensation insures that medical professionals will find it more economically advantageous to avoid future careless injuries to patients than to keep paying damage awards.

If I believed this—if I believed there were enough money in the world to accomplish this—I know I would sue in an irregular heartbeat.

I confer with a colleague who is a torts professor. She has already urged me to sue, but I want to ask her about the possibility of change at the famous cancer center. Would a lawsuit be an actual deterrent? Or would the cancer center, now a defendant, simply circle the wagons as I'd seen other defendants do, not changing policies, practices or personnel lest this be viewed as an admission of wrongdoing. She is less than hopeful about the prospects of reform.

I finally consult an attorney. Reputed to be the best "med-mal" attorney in the state and by fortuity employing one of my former students.

My former student is pleased to see me.

Alive.

"When I heard what you had, I thought for sure you were a goner."

Obviously, it is not only members of the medical profession who could benefit from an infusion of compassion.

Or at least tact.

She excitedly tells me about an eight-million-dollar settlement for a patient whose stomach was wrongly removed.

I become dizzy and nauseous. My throat burns and my mind recedes. I must look pale, because she offers me a chair.

When she asks me how I am, I respond that I am great. Fine. Recovered completely.

We review the medical records.

"You should see a heart specialist so we can determine the permanent damage. And a neurologist for nerve damage. Do you have any symptoms?"

No. No. No. No. No. No.

She frowns.

An airtight case on liability, no difficulties there. But we need some permanent damages to make the case more lucrative.

"You look good with short hair," she says as I leave.

Just as I researched my cancer, leading me to the out-of-network doctors, I research malpractice, hoping I will be led to a decision.

The failure to diagnose. The lost chance doctrine, allowing some recovery for terminally ill patients. Community or national standards of care. The constitutionality of damages cap statutes. *Res Ipsa Loquitur.* The admissibility of certain hospital records. The enforcement of a gag order.

What would my gag order provide?

That I, as a condition of settlement, agree

not to publicly criticize the defendant doctors, medical personnel, or organization, or anyone associated therewith,

not to disclose the terms of the settlement either privately or publicly,

and not to publish or cause to be published any work related to the litigation or the events underlying the litigation, in any form or manner whatsoever, in perpetuity.

To agree—forever—not to talk or write about what happened to me is more unthinkable than what happened to me.

I will not be silent.

I will not be sick.

I let the statute of limitations lapse.

I celebrate by going out to dinner.

How wonderful the food tastes.

How lucid the conversation.

How good not to be a case, legal or medical, difficult or otherwise.

But I live with this terrible knowledge: that if I had been a little less stubborn, a little more awed by authority, a little less economically privileged, a little more charmed by tranquilizers, a little less able to research my own disease, or simply unlucky, I'd be dead now.

And you would not be reading this.

Case closed.

•

Rutbann Robson is a Professor of Law at the City University of New York School of Law and has written widely on lesbian legal theory, including Sappho Goes to Law School *(Columbia University Press, 1998). She is the author of several novels, including* A/K/A *(St. Martin's Press, 1998).*

The Agony and the Agony

Deborah McDonald

∽

The plan was to break open the tiny tabernacle, split the relic, swallow it and see what transpired. To carry out this borderline sacrilegious project, though it was not our intent to be irreverent in any way, we used one of mother's steel steak knives, carefully dissecting the microscopic sliver of St. Therese's shinbone, no bigger than a pinhead, easier than swallowing half a baby aspirin. For verification and camaraderie as much as anything, I enlisted my sister Michele, thirteen months younger than I, herself a saint in training. Michele and I looked at each other and gulped.

The repercussions were overwhelmingly uneventful. We wore ourselves weary during the ensuing weeks waiting for a more powerful moment: a rainbow above our house on Konzier Drive, say, or maybe a rose suddenly blooming out of season. That's the way it was in *Fifteen Saints for Girls*, the book that had riled me up and launched my youthful fanaticism, pain and miracles somehow provocatively entwined. Therese of Lisieux, known as "The Little Flower," was my favorite. Born in France to a wealthy family, the youngest of nine children, she had rejected worldly pleasures and entered the contemplative order of Carmelite nuns at age fifteen, then died of tuberculosis at twenty-four. Her spiritual journey included hair shirts and self-inflicted . pain—like soap bubbles through a wand, images as profound as they were confusing to an eight-year-old zealot.

Giving up chocolate bars for Lent seemed paltry by comparison, the measly sacrifice of a spoiled, post-Depression kid whose level of suffering had yet to exceed summer mosquito bites, easily negated by Dad, who paid five cents per welt.

It was during this phase of my girlhood that Uncle Tom—really a second cousin and a priest—gave me an authentic relic of St. Therese, a microscopic piece of her shinbone enshrined in an ornate filigree case shaped like a sun, studded with red rubies, complete with official Vatican papers. "Gross," pronounced one of my best friends as we'd sit for hours looking out the window, listening to my transistor radio. But I was trapped by the sheer possession of something so supernatural.

And there was the imagined epigraph, unrevealed but significantly looming. My complete conviction that miracles could happen to even the most ordinary of girls, a repetitive tenet of the saintly biographies, was neurally linked in my developing mind to the concept of the American Indian shaman, who used to uncover the medicinal powers of plants and herbs by slowly exposing himself to an unknown plant substance in tiny increments—first his skin, then lightly touching it to his tongue, then finally ingesting a minuscule tidbit. It became infinitely clear that the path to enlightenment was plausible.

One unexpected development. Along with initiating "The Plan," I quickly realized my ominous conjecture justified the necessity of losing the gold case. Mortals were far too attached to material goods, I rationalized, not to mention that sooner or later, Mother was bound to ask about the relic. If she never saw it, we'd significantly cut our chances of discovery. Telling a lie could defeat our good intentions. Even worse, it might make the whole thing a sin. I was still swinging on grapevines and hadn't yet developed the worldly foresight to consider that a couple of those rubies might have fed a small country.

We buried the case at the bottom of the kitchen trash.

By the time Mother rang the dinner bell that night, "The Plan" was beginning to seem more like a Wally and Beaver caper than a heavenly prospectus. I felt a stab of guilt, terror even. Had I really thought the whole thing through? My list of fears compounded as the days wore on with no miracles on the horizon, but to protect Michele, the innocent victim of my overanxious quest for holiness, I kept these to myself.

I shrugged off the idea of an instant miracle—I hadn't actually asked for anything specifically—and decided to evaluate the situation as one might evaluate a fortune cookie limerick pasted hopefully on a refrigerator door. That is, see if anything struck as the days passed.

The supernatural had a surrealist stratagem sans mortal control. Sure. Miracles could take days, maybe weeks? Miracles might require patience. Pilgrims to Lourdes and Fatima were often healed spontaneously, but they had made draconian journeys in wheelchairs and on stretchers, I reasoned, and deserved instant gratification. Christ raised Lazarus from the dead in an instant, but he had a mere thirty-three years on the planet to complete a mission that would have to last until Armageddon.

Meanwhile, I came up with Plan II to circumvent any hazy wrongdoing regarding the first. Michele and I would scour the daily newspaper, point to a name in the obituaries and pray for that person all day. It seemed a worthy project, something the Little Flower might have done. *Fifteen Saints for Girls* said her glory was making differences in small ways. I took the name Theresa for my Confirmation in her honor, and because I wanted to be commensurably holy, I waited for pain.

I got the flu that year and had to miss New Year's dinner at Uncle Ed's, ham studded with cloves, scalloped potatoes, fancy chocolates and cashews. My fever was so high I secretly hoped it was all part of being divinely tested. Mother and Dad let me lie in their mahogany bed and watch TV, which wasn't so bad really. I wondered if that even counted as pain. Michele got hit in the head with a rock by Chuckie Gerson playing cowboys and Indians and had to have stitches in her scalp. That counted for her.

Mother never quizzed me once about the missing relic—an astonishing enough miracle in and of itself.

The idea of hotly awaited, saintly pain thinned with time and boys. I became consumed with how to make myself look more like Cher than the Little Flower. I started reading Allen Ginsberg and dating a Vietnam war resister who drove an MG with only one door. It was the Sixties. St. Therese's shinbone story had metamorphosed into good coffeehouse satire while retaining a stoic and admirable legacy during the peace movement years. Sometimes, when I'd see some odd thing in a thrift store or an antique emporium, I'd wish I still had that exquisite gold case.

If you could escape your fate, whose life would you step into? Put all lives in one basket and you'd most likely choose your own. I was plagued with colitis in my twenties but it went into remission. I was divorced but fell madly in love again. My children were intelligent, healthy, fun. I went back to college when they were teenagers, graduated with a degree in journalism, bought my first house, got my first writing job. Just when life seemed, relatively speaking, wonderful, a strange, crushing pain began to shoot down my arm in a most inhumane fashion. My neck and back muscles went into severe spasm, more like flagstone than flesh. Doctors and surgeons sighed at the pathology of my spine. It made sense for a football player or a world class wrestler, not a food critic with a taste for relics. Pain had become a snotty child playing an endless game of tag, intent on driving me away from the things I loved most.

Five years down the road, I am madly spilling my papers around four A.M., searching for an 800 number copied from a late night infomercial for a miracle cream called "Blue Stuff." I am in desperate pain. In the cerebral world, anything called "Blue Stuff," advertised when all but bartenders and shift workers are asleep, sounds nonsensical, but in the world of pain, where short-term memory is a casualty, touting an anesthetic as "Blue Stuff" seems completely logical. I wouldn't wake up and be able to recall, say, a product called "Apocalypse Now." I might remember that it had a name like a movie that started with an "A." But "Blue Stuff," I could remember that. And forty dollars? A price just high enough to make one stop and consider, "Is this a rip-off or a theatrical tour de force to cover up a clandestine cure?" It's barely a bag of groceries. In the light of day, more pain, less hope. I'm still looking for that damn piece of paper.

Did I ever pray for pain? C'mon. I was just a kid. I never meant to, and if I did, claiming youth, I take it back.

∾

I should confess that Prior to Pain, I maintained a legacy of resisting support group types. As far back as high school, I refused to join National Honor Society and declined having my picture taken for the senior yearbook. Those touched-up photos looked more like a funeral pose than the portrait of a young girl who wore love beads and McCarthy buttons. It was the late Sixties and it all seemed so narcissistic when you had friends who were going to prison instead of Vietnam, others coming home in body bags. I was trying to stay out of the high school limelight and avoiding the Trivial at all costs.

Pain starts like a war, a surprise aggressor taking victims in open revolt during the night. You become the defenseless transgressed. It strikes; you fight. At first you're in shock, struggling for equilibrium. I had no perception of fear in the beginning. Just fight. Violent retaliation. Fear creeps in as the pain fails to subside, and as its intensity grows, so does its cruelty. After two years of battle, with muscles locked in perpetual spasm, persistent pain keeping me from the things I loved most, enough physical therapy that my insurance company informed me I was close to reaching my "lifetime" limit, I decided to join a Pain Group.

"You'll never come back," I remember Russell, a longtime regular, saying after my first foray into the Pain Group, and I knew this was meant as a challenge. I was a cynical smart aleck that first session, firing questions at the doctor, hammering away at the biology of pain, determined to uncover any secrets being kept from me, somewhere in France probably, at places where the movie stars and people with money go for cures. Run-down and isolated for so long, I was surprised by my reemerging spunk. With something new to liquefy the loneliness, I couldn't wait for six o'clock on Thursdays.

Somehow, a clinical room in an overlit hospital became our secret club. We'd turn the lights down low, fix each other cups of tea, trade books and tapes, weird supplements, secrets for pain-jolting, middle-of-the-night meltdowns. We were held together in combat.

My comrades in pain gasped when I said I didn't pray. I didn't take prayer literally, that is, I didn't perceive it as one-on-one connection at a bargaining table between a divine entity and a creature like myself. But because of them I began a ritual conversation I call praying. I wish for small things, mostly short periods of relief. A year? Six months? Could I just get that? Every other day? Give it to me every other day. Break it into half a day? Sometimes I sneak in asking for a good night's sleep. Sometimes I make vows. "I'll do something that really matters. I'll go to hospitals and sit with people in dim rooms who need me." Of course, I strike bargains, make promises. "Just take the damn pain away and I'll carry placards for research, start marathons for money, fight the nonsense about banning pain medications because they are being used as street drugs." Sometimes, I just think, "Oh please give everyone a few days of real, unrelenting pain," and then I can't help but pick out a particular nemesis or two, something Therese of Lisieux would have flogged herself bloody for. And then my Catholic schoolgirl guilt invades my conscience and I apologize. I ask for the pain I had back in 1999. That would be fine.

One of my physical therapists meditates early in the morning, and in one of these moments, it came to her that I should peck on my computer while sitting on one of those giant, inflatable exercise balls. She ordered one according to the length of my legs, and other than when I have to make a deadline, in which case I seem to need the same hard stool I've always sat on, I use the ball. It's a pretty inane picture if you step back and take it in. Regardless of ergonomics, I am able to write less and less.

I fail to grasp the hypocrisy that glamorizes silent suffering. I have little patience for false bravado. Why are people who suffer quietly supposedly the "good people"? I've thought of blaming Jackie Kennedy somewhere in there (even Jesus cried out from the cross) but I know that's not fair. Jackie rightfully held herself together bravely for the nation during the dark days following her husband's assassination. But when she was dying of cancer, behind the dark glasses and head scarves, I hope she cried. I really do. People came right up to Jesus and begged for pain relief. They moaned. They cried. He never told them to buck up and be silent. He placed his hands on them.

"There are no bridges to let anyone in on the dragons of your private pain world," says my husband Brad, who has had Crohn's disease since he was twenty and knows something about getting sick when your life is just ahead of you. Brad was a college student, a history major, a drummer, when he started having embarrassing gastrointestinal symptoms—painful bloating, cramping, gas. He had never heard of Crohn's disease. His descent into illness involved a year of undiagnosed symptoms. Just stress, maybe ulcers. Watch your diet, he was told. The pain kept escalating, but of course, you can't see pain. Barium eventually revealed Crohn's disease.

The term "incurable" rang in his head. He graduated from college a term early, took a job, all the while growing sicker and sicker. Finally, he took a month off. Two months later, he could barely walk or eat. Three weeks after that, he started vomiting black gruel. His bowel had a pinhole perforation but the doctors hadn't discovered it with all the fine-tuned testing. They forced an NG (nasal gut) tube down his throat. "They hold you down, your eyes tear up, you feel like you'll choke to death. In retrospect, I've had good people do it, and I've had beginners—and believe me, you don't want a beginner."

Your body creates about a quart of gastrointestinal fluids each day if you are properly hydrated, even if you don't eat, so emptying his bowels eased the pain and the perforation remained undetected. After ten days they pulled the tube. Spying a cracker on his hospital neighbor's tray, he snuck two bites. The cracker turned out to be the proverbial straw—13–14 inches of weakened intestine split open within the time it took the Saltine to travel the length of his small bowel.

He got out two yelps before his right side became paralyzed. "I didn't need anybody to tell me I was dying. At that point, you simply don't care. You just want it to stop." Only about 3 percent of Crohn's patients ever rupture. But rupturing a second time? Doctors say it just doesn't happen.

When it did almost twenty years later, I was at work. Brad had been going downhill steadily for months. During a presurgical consult at Cleveland Clinic, it had been determined that he had to have more small bowel removed. I flinched, asking the specialist to refer us to a Pittsburgh gastroenterologist, "just in case." When you live with someone with a chronic illness, the "what if" syndrome is a life preserver. "What if we didn't have time to Life-Flight him to Cleveland if something went wrong before the prescheduled surgery? What if . . ."

Brad was so weak that he resisted another doctor visit, but I dragged him anyway. The doctor in Pittsburgh, trained by the famed surgeon from Cleveland, sat knee-to-knee with Brad, looking him right in the eye—little things that can make doctors welcomingly human. He reviewed his films carefully, agreed that surgery was imminent. As we left, he mentioned that we were his last patients that day, that he was off on a long-awaited vacation with his wife. I tucked his card into my coat pocket. "Bon voyage," I said, shaking his hand. "I *like* him," Brad managed to croak.

I went off to work, leaving Brad in his world of pain. Shortly after I arrived, the telephone rang. "You better come home," Brad squeaked. On the street, I could hear him through the thick stone walls of our old house, a deadly, haunting wail. He emerged from the garbage can long enough to call out, "I've ruptured."

I phoned 911, pulled the doctor's card out of my coat pocket. "He's gone," the secretary barked. "*Gone.* He doesn't even have his pager." I garbled my number anyway. As the ambulance came roaring up the drive, the phone rang. "I'll meet you at the ER," the doctor said. The memory of the relic flickered as my focus dissolved. The miracle was slightly imperfect, however. Brad was forced to spend the night writhing in pain because, though the good doctor stayed behind, most likely pissing off his wife, not to mention saving Brad's life, he delayed operating, not thinking it possible that Brad had ruptured a second time. I saw pain that night I hope never to see again.

"You have been given the opportunity to experience chronic pain," began a Cleveland Clinic spine specialist as he walked into the room after reviewing my MRIs. I slumped lower into my chair, stared at the ceiling. This, I had discovered, had become the latest buzz-phrase, a hip approach in the mode of psychobabble when you can't retrieve the patient from the pit back to the natural world. The nouveau way of lowering the boom, direct but pseudo–Far Eastern. If only I had a baseball bat, I imagined, I could take a swing at his kneecap and then calmly, clinically, with perfect, detached professionalism, recite his lines back to him.

Again, I apologize to the deity.

I wanted to ask about Norman Cousins, ascorbic acid IVs, Andrew Weil, hyperbaric chambers, intramuscular Botox, subcutaneous administration of growth hormone. An experimental pain drug that doesn't turn your brain blotto?

Instead, I gave him the look I used to give my mother when I was sixteen, then talked about him loudly when he left the room, knowing he could hear me. He was nicer when he came back, with literature to quiet me down, offering me an extended stay we both knew my insurance wouldn't pay for. We even got friendly for a moment, engaged in light banter. I asked him to direct us to a restaurant, envisioning him swirling an after-work cocktail with a colleague, flushing the day's case residue out of his system.

People tend to shun the ugliness of pain, partly because it makes onlookers feel helpless, depressed, but mostly because they realize there's nothing but sheer luck between themselves and a similar fate. Pain research will never escalate if those of us who are in pain don't rail. Why don't we? Because we're afraid. Powerless. You quickly become marginalized if you complain. The reasons are as ambiguous as they are complex, but I can tell you there's a constant low humming in the back of our minds that keeps us silent—whatever relief we've been granted may be taken away. Practitioners have to navigate a maze of insurance issues and puritanical drug regulations distracting them from the metaphysical and ethical issues of pain management. We're sent to pain clinics that are closing their doors and sending us back to the primary care doctors who sent us there in the first place. Doctors may mistake our pain for hysteria and write us off as malcontents. Lucky you are to find a doctor who has suffered severe pain, either chronically or acutely, because the subject matter is given scant attention in medical training. The rights of the ill have been so trampled down by the "War on Drugs" that the legitimate patient who needs pain medication has to jump through such laborious hoops that I've heard eighty-year-old women in pharmacy lines say they are treated like street addicts.

∽

New Year's Eve. Instead of making a last-minute stop for a bottle of bubbly, I sat in an outpatient hospital room for about eight hours, waiting for a doctor to enter my neck with a needle, cauterizing nerves. I had been told not to take my muscle relaxants. As a result, my neck was like a stone pillar. The doctor kept coming around, engaging in rather lengthy discussions. The more we talked the less we liked each other, and the less we liked each other, the more reluctant I was to surrender to the procedure. I was waffling up until the last moment, chickening out, recanting, back and forth, something loose inside of me clawing away at a gut feeling of impending doom. When I was finally wheeled into the operating room, stuck on a gurney big enough for a skinny midget, strapped down, given no anesthetic, I was trembling. Of sound mind sans medication, I distinctly remember being told, "Call out if you feel any pain." The needle went in, blocked by spasm.

I gasped when the pain caught me by surprise, as I'd been instructed. The doctor ripped off his rubber gloves, aborting the procedure. I called faintly after him, "Please, let's try again. I'll try again." But he was off, down the hall with a plastic model of the spine, expounding with great rancor. My husband said he could not make out much of the heady medical jargon, but that the doctor resembled a man engaged in damage control in the spin room of a political campaign.

Meanwhile, half naked and out of options, I felt small, lost, abandoned, Hester Prynne in a roomful of gawking residents, a scarlet letter on my chest. I hung my head, dressed and slumped in one of the vinyl hospital lobby chairs waiting for the car. And I started to cry. And cry. It was New Year's Eve and I cried because there were so many people behind those walls just hanging on for their next dose. I cried for Brad all over again, for kids all over the world uprooted from childhood by pain. I cried because Jackie Kennedy didn't. I cried for all the choking eulogies praising silent suffering. I cried because I find silence demeaning, not courageous. I cried because I am in too much pain to sit at the computer and browse the Internet to figure out if somewhere, someone has found something I haven't tried. I cried because my muscles were slamming into my spine like a wrecking ball and "Blue Stuff" didn't work.

Can I remember what it was like *not* to have pain, a hypnotist asked me the other day. I stopped for a moment. "Yeah, I do," I said like an overeager bride. "*I do.*"

"Then I can help you," she said. "But not today." My expression fell harder than a kid who had just lost heaping double scoops from the top of a sugar cone. "Next week I may have an opening." She pulled out her smooth leather appointment book. "Of course, my services are not covered by insurance. The fee is ninety dollars, payable at the end of each session."

•

Deborah McDonald grew up in Pittsburgh during the 1950s. She is a freelance writer and food critic.

Burden of Oath

Linda Peeno, MD

ᴄ

I will use regimens for the benefit of the ill
In accordance with my ability
And my judgment,
But from what is to their harm or injustice
I will keep them . . .
In a pure and holy way
I will guard my life and my techne . . .
Into as many houses as I may enter,
I will go for the benefit of the ill.[1]

A ninety-year-old man died, an event that wouldn't prompt many of us to take a second glance at the obituaries. Yet I spent eight hours today trying to explain a grim chain of events leading to this death. The harder I struggled to weave meaning, the more a lawyer, representing a large health insurance company, attempted to unravel it. In many ways, we simply played a chess game of words. Except I was under oath.

I attempted to reconstruct the events of the man's last days through a deposition, a legal procedure theoretically designed to reveal and challenge an expert's opinions in a lawsuit. As a physician with special knowledge about the inner workings of the health industry, I practice a kind of medicine Hippocrates never could have imagined. Instead of potions and procedures, my care of patients requires language and analysis.

I sit now at my kitchen table, a place of refuge. I should *do* something—eat, read mail, return calls, work—but the late afternoon sun presses across my chair, and the heat of the day immobilizes me. I can see tips of trees through the kitchen window. An early spring breeze ruffles them, causing speckles of light and shadow to flicker on the floor. I should open some windows and doors for air. But the slant of the late sun saddens me. With the day's end, I feel overwhelmed by all that's left undone.

I spent three days preparing for the deposition, reading and analyzing thousands of pages of documents. Last night I had only a few hours of sleep, waking early to work more. I always fear I will forget something critical from a contract, policy or testimony. But all that preparation seems futile now. The lawyer just spent hours dissecting my personal and professional life. The process was less about the facts of the patient's death, and more about intimidating me. The lawyer adeptly upended so much of what I had done, turned work about which I was pleased into something that appeared to be a failure, turned writings over which I had agonized into something for which I should be apologetic.

Why do this, I wonder.

It takes special knowledge to articulate long threads of casual connections between inappropriate cost-cutting and harmful patient care. My job demands painstaking exploration of whole systems most others ignore, discount, or just don't understand. I see firsthand the ways we have created a health system unprecedented in its ill effects. Patients now suffer not only from their diseases, but also from the *management* of their diseases.

Although I can do little now for the man who died, I can help identify patterns of practice that risk harming other patients. Patients such as this man are evidence of processes gone tragically awry, but their stories are all too often dismissed as "mere anecdotes"—the health industry's means of explaining away responsibility. Yet when we understand the ways corporations affect patient care, we can potentially provide corrections—

a nice, simple ideal that caused me to change my work as a physician several years ago. Now I work full-time assisting attorneys, policymakers and members of the public who try to gain correctives and recompense for people who have been or who are at risk of being abused by a system that puts profits over patient care.

When I first testified in a case against an HMO, I believed naively that public knowledge and legal accountability would change the actions of health-care companies. Now, more than five years and fifty cases later, the only difference I see is in the increased subtlety of harm, in the ever more inventive elusion of responsibility. My house is a vault of suppressed information, an inaccessible archive of documents protected by sealed confidentiality orders and settlement agreements.

Today the lawyer referred repeatedly to the patient as just a "ninety-year-old man, wheelchair-bound, with dementia"—suggesting, it seemed, that his age and condition justified the poor care he had received. I finally asked her directly if her characterization meant that the patient was too old and sick to deserve either the expense—or hope—of care. She feigned outrage at my accusation, but I was haunted through the entire deposition by the thought that this man had become *disposable.*

There are, of course, other persons, including some physicians, who would argue that such a man—that anyone sufficiently old and sufficiently sick—should receive a different kind of care, though they would never of course admit to using those criteria. Some would justify their position with claims of kindness: why should we subject someone like this to prolonged life? Others would claim that it is necessary rationing: we can redirect dollars spent on potentially futile care to those who need it more—children, for example. These arguments sound rational in the abstract. But with particular patients, their fallacies multiply: acts of so-called kindness can become ruses for cost-cutting, and savings from denials go not to needier patients, but more often to hungrier bottom lines.

Medicine is inherently *particular,* as Dr. Francis Peabody once told Harvard medical students. One essential quality of the clinician, according to Dr. Peabody, is interest in humanity, for the secret of the care of patients is in caring for *the* patient. If we do not keep specific patients—particular human beings—in mind in our systems of care, we can become the causes, however remote, of cost accounting masked as beneficence, and harm masked as utility. We then perpetuate our peculiarly American brand of health delivery, the only health system that rations care for the financial benefit of those who are supposed to provide that care.

Today the lawyer avoided all my attempts to individualize the patient. The man, although ninety, had been living at home alone. His son described him as clear-thinking and independent. After a fall, he went to his doctor with a complaint of pain in his leg. Even though an X-ray confirmed a fractured hip, and a note by the radiologist indicated the patient would be transported to the hospital for surgery, another document showed that some unidentifiable person canceled the admission. The doctor sent the patient home instead, and ordered an evaluation by Hospice, the one treatment in this case that cost the doctor and health plan nothing—a benefit of their astute cost-shifting.

A Hospice nurse promptly told the doctor that the patient's nonterminal condition made him ineligible for Hospice care. So the patient suffered for several days at home, without assistance, pain medications or treatment for the fracture. As the pain worsened, the family pleaded with the doctor to admit the man to the hospital. Mysteriously, the patient acquired another diagnosis at the time of his admission: the doctor said he suffered from "dementia," something unsupported by other medical records, previous living conditions or history provided by the son.

Two days after the doctor finally performed surgery on the hip fracture, he sent the patient to a nursing home for rehabilitation and physical therapy. When the patient arrived there, he already had bedsores from his hospitalization. Despite his medical needs, no doctor saw him during his week in the nursing home. A physical therapist told the doctor and the insurance company that the patient could not do therapy or rehabilitation without a special medical device to relieve pressure from the sores on his heels. A document in the records showed that someone first approved the device, but then deleted that approval before sending the request to the equipment company. A note found in the documents explained that the doctor objected to the cost, although it was less than three hundred dollars. One is left to wonder if the doctor and insurance company thought that even a few hundred dollars was too much to spend on a man they believed moved closer every day to death.

The doctor, who had not seen the patient in the several days since his discharge from the hospital, sent the patient home after giving an order by telephone. At first, the doctor did not arrange home health care, but when family members pleaded again for help, home health nurses were allowed to visit. When the nurses complained about the increasingly infected, deepening wounds, the doctor responded, not with hospitalization, but with a discontinuation of home health care.

After receiving reports about worsening of the bedsores, the doctor made a house call, something that would, under other circumstances, signify an unusually caring physician. But this doctor didn't go because he cared so much; he went because he cared so little—he simply hoped to save the cost of a hospitalization. There at the patient's house, with the patient in his own bed, the doctor performed surgery—without proper instruments, and without anesthesia. With the patient writhing and screaming in bed, the doctor scraped rotting flesh down to the muscle and bone—living tissue that bled and registered pain.

After more pleading from the family, the doctor finally sent the patient back to the hospital. Later the man died from a massive infection caused by progressive, untreated pressure wounds.

I know there are persons who would argue that, at most, this was a case of physician negligence, or that the physician couldn't have prevented what happened, since the man was going to die anyway. The claim for inevitable death is a favorite among insurance companies. However, some particulars cannot be ignored.

Unbeknownst to the patient or his family, the primary care physician and the insurance company had a financial arrangement by which they each received bonuses when allotted money wasn't spent on medical care. This operated according to simple arithmetic: spend less, make more. Furthermore, when doctors spent too much, they not only lost money, they risked deficits that would require them to pay penalties to the insurance company.

Maybe this arrangement had no effect on the decisions and outcome, as the insurance company argues. Or if it did, the insurance company is not responsible for how a doctor practices—another favorite argument. Some court of law or public opinion should consider if these financial arrangements resulted in a chain of deadly decisions for this man, a chain in which every point marked a cost-cutting choice without regard for the patient. The people of this country—every one a potential patient in such a system—should be allowed to determine if this is an isolated case, or if it is the logical result of a health-care system in urgent need of correction.

My funk increases as the room darkens. The last light is a smudge of red just behind the lacy branches of the trees I can see. A faint rose glow now lights the room just beyond the kitchen. From my chair, I can see four boxes on the dining room floor—a new case. I groan, feeling oppressed as much by the burden of work that they represent as by the heat. As the boxes melt away into the darkening room, I realize how sick I am of this health-care mess. I am sick of the fight, sick of the increasing sophistication of the health indus- try's dereliction of duty, sick of witnessing needless suffering, and most of all, sick of feeling impotent to make any real change.

My house overflows with paper—evidence of a monstrous change in medicine, something we now call "managed care." When I graduated from medical school in 1978, the term didn't exist in my vocabulary. Now I have more than two hundred books about the subject. Piles of "managed care" documents—benefit books, policy and procedure manuals, contracts, financial reports, marketing materials, corporate communications, utilization and qual- ity profiles—litter rooms once filled only with books on philosophy, literature, science and theology. I have read more of these documents than any person I know in this country. I tire of the health-care industry's failed promises and the damage it does to patients. I shudder when I think that Hippocrates binds me to a three-thousand-year-old oath outlining a way of life, not just the treatment of patients. These are words that take root, ground me.

Thirty years ago, almost to this day, a young family doctor begged me to apply to medical school. I had seen him a few times for simple ailments, typical colds and sore throats. One day, as I sat on his exam table, trying to describe a new, but vague, illness, he stood back and asked directly: what is really wrong?

I burst into tears. I had just received a letter denying me admission to nursing school, a path I believed would always assure work so I could support my daughter and still pursue graduate work in philosophy. The head of the nursing school told me that the program was too demanding for a single mother with a small baby. Fortunately, upon hearing my story, my doctor spent time asking questions rather than doing tests, and what he prescribed was far more powerful than any drug.

A few days later, when I returned for a second visit, he told me he had been thinking about our conversation. Forget nursing school, he said. You should go to medical school. I have this vision, he went on, of you walking in a crisp white coat down a sunlit hall of a hospital.

Years later, long fluorescent tubes, not the sun, lit the halls I walked. My white coat turned dingy with wear, and often hung limp after long hours of work. No day in my life as a doctor ever manifested the scene the way my doctor imagined it, but I carried that image—his ideal—through the hard years of training, my balm for fear, fatigue, doubt and despair.

At one point, the perfect image of that clean, bright hall blurred with a vision of a darker place. It came one hot afternoon. I had walked off a ward and turned down a long corridor, on my way to tell a mother about the death of her son. The oppressive heat had driven everyone to cooler places, and my steps echoed through the emptiness of the long hall. I walked as slowly as possible, at first to delay my encounter with the mother, and then to soften the sounds of the steps that magnified my loneliness. I longed for the hall to have no end and to make no sound.

As I walked, an image came to me. I was in another large hall, dimly lit and packed with people. All around me, people stood, sat or moved in and out of groups. Some laughed. Some whined or cried. Some were quiet, and others moved about frenetically. Some begged for help. Others tended to their needs. Periodically a door would open, and a name would be called. One by one, individuals exited the room and did not return.

The young boy who had just died had become a favorite patient. His disease and eventual death seemed inexplicable. I could think of nothing to tell his mother. Maybe this is just what life is like, I thought, as I imagined that hall filled with people. We pass through this room briefly, marking time until our name is called. Then we leave. Maybe that is all there is.

The sky is now so dark the trees are no longer visible. I have a fleeting urge to leave the house and walk to those imperceptible masses just to touch their trunks.

Today the lawyer spent nearly an hour asking questions about a patient whose death I caused. While working for an insurance company in 1987, I denied a man a life-saving procedure. It took years for me to understand what I had done, because an act of honest confession is unacceptable to the business of health care. The lawyer circled the issue round and round, attempting to break apart my words and feelings until they were meaningless and empty.

A young man caught what seemed to be a simple cold. Instead, he had a virus that attacked his heart, leaving him no hope of recovery without a heart transplant. After critical weeks had passed, a hospital in another state had a donor. While teams of surgical personnel prepared for the surgery, a clerk in the hospital's admissions department placed a call to our insurance company for authorization. A nurse at the company took the call, but could not give medical approval for the case. She referred it to the doctor in charge of "medical review."

I was that doctor, part of a new breed of medical professionals far removed from the bedside. I made decisions about the "medical necessity" of procedures that other physicians requested for their patients. Though new to me, this sort of work was generously reimbursed and quite easy compared to the physically exhausting work in an emergency room, the usual place for a moonlighting physician. No one questioned how it was possible for a physician distant from a patient and without the requesting physician's clinical knowledge and experience to make appropriate medical decisions, especially when those decisions altered a patient's course of care.

Although I had been working for only a few months, I was already familiar with the unspoken prime requirement of the job: Save the company as much money as possible. Most of the cases referred to physicians like me were more "economic" than "medical." More than once, my superior, also a physician, paid me visits to discuss the nature of my job and the decisions I made. I was told frequently that my medical degree helped give medical justification to economic decisions. He never failed to remind me that, in contrast to other work I might do as a physician, I was now an *employee* of a company, which, in case I should forget, issued my paycheck.

When the request for the heart transplant came to me, I thought my task was simple. Since we made determinations about medical necessity, I didn't understand why I had the case. Surely no physician would perform a medically *unnecessary* heart transplant. Believing it was a mistake, I simply called the transplant surgeon, documented the medical history and authorized the procedure.

Just as I started to stamp "APPROVE" on the request, a nurse burst into the office to tell me that I must call the surgeon back. We have a way to deny the case, she said. The benefits department discovered an exclusion for heart transplants in this man's contract.

With clear grounds for a technical denial, I called the surgeon to tell him we would not pay for the transplant. At first he couldn't believe it. He spat questions through the phone: How could we sell contracts like that? How did this man get on a transplant list and get to the hospital if his contract was so clear? Even if the contract was right, how could we deny him at this point? *Don't you realize, Dr. Peeno, that you have issued this man a death sentence?*

In the fury of the moment, these questions didn't register. I had just saved my company a half-million dollars. Later that day, the Vice President for Medical Affairs complimented me on my good work, and assured me that I had finally grasped the nature of my professional responsibilities as a physician with the company. My fellow physician reviewers envied my moment of success.

Initially I felt a kind of confidence about my actions. I fulfilled the expectations of my job. We had a contract and could legitimately enforce it. Our country suffered from escalating health-care costs that required us to limit expenditures. But a few days later, as I walked through the company's marble rotunda, I saw a new sculpture—a piece that I eventually discovered cost $3.8 million dollars, eight times the price of a heart transplant.

What had I done? I began to feel something deep but ill-defined, a sense of unnamable dread. I finally couldn't ignore reality: I participated in a young man's death by performing well a job I never questioned. Although everything about the new organization of health care conspired to diminish my sense of connection to the man, and though his initial facelessness diminished my sense of responsibility, I couldn't shake his presence.

Now, the world through the kitchen window is solid black, everything folded together. The heat from the day's sun, still trapped in my closed house, makes me miserable, yet I still cannot find the energy to move. Leaving my chair means a return to work, a return to the burden of an oath and a profession I continue to question.

Several weeks ago, I began reading a new philosophy book, essays by a French philosopher named Emmanuel Levinas. He writes about the primacy of the *other*, embodied, he believes, in the face-to-face experience. Responsibility, for Levinas, is not just our answer for that which we have originated, but commands that we answer even for situations we did not bring about. We are responsible, he claims, not only for our own deeds, but also for the deeds of others. It's a heavy burden, I think, but one that I realize has underpinned my evolving view of life and work as both a physician and a human being.

Some are guilty, says Jewish theologian Abraham Joshua Heschel, but all are responsible. Yet we live in a culture that makes us masters at eluding responsibility, even when the cause-effect chain of actions and responses seems direct and obvious. How easy it is to claim ignorance, impotence, indecision, incompetence, or any number of other mitigating conditions. And, of course, the easiest plea in a culture of legislation, administrative rules and professional codes is simply to say, *I* am not *required* to do this.

Levinas says to know a fellow person is not to thematize him or her as an object, but to *greet* the person. This requires an encounter, a kind of *welcoming* that binds us inextricably to all the individuals about us. Our fellow persons are not mere objects of perception, but persons who make appeals and require responses. An encounter, according to Levinas, can never be complete or total. There is always a surplus of available action: I can always do more. I create continuous conditions of possibility, and every decision I make is not only about what action to take, but also about what kind of person I want to be.

My work as a physician—even a physician who now only uses words as my tools for healing—is inherently linked to patients, real human beings who command something of me. These persons, with whom I have an unbreak-able relationship, make demands of me, for they always have, as Levinas argues, a *face*—even if I do not physically see it. Because of the work I do now as a physician, I must struggle harder to give *presence* to patients, especially those made distant and abstract by the medical and legal systems. I must bring them close enough to disturb me and to disturb others too. To *hear their cries*, as Levinas writes.

To claim that kind of responsibility is to seek more, not less, as Hippocrates no doubt meant when he wrote the Hippocratic Oath. For all the frustration, the hours spent reading documents, the meetings with lawyers, the exhausting cross-country flights to depositions and trials, my life and work are intertwined in ways that ultimately make both richer. My oaths—medical and legal—require a way of being as well as doing, a way of acting as well as speaking. Yes, I risk—and experience—futility. But maybe the antidote lies in seeking out increasingly longer, more complex chains of interrelationships and responsibility, and understanding that what sometimes appears futile may just be the result of views which are still too narrow, and on which too little light has been shed.

With this thought, I get up from my chair and get on with things. I must eat, read mail, return calls, work. I have four new boxes to open. First, though, the house needs fresh air. When I open the kitchen window, a cool breeze blows through, and I see that the trees are now backlit by a clear, bright moon.

•

Linda Peeno *is a physician whose sole patient is our seriously ill health-care system. Her experience as a medical reviewer for a prominent HMO was the subject of* Damaged Care, *a television movie. Most recently, she was featured in* The New York Times. *When she's not writing, speaking, or consulting on ethical issues in health care, she can be found in Louisville, Kentucky, reading, planning her next mountaineering adventure, or helping to develop the mind, heart, and spirit of her new granddaughter.*

---

1. Heinrich Von Staden, "'In a pure and holy way': Personal and Professional Conduct in the Hippocratic Oath," *Journal of the History of Medicine and Allied Sciences* 51 (1996): 406–408.

Babies as a Problem

Richard Beach

∾

There's an extra spring in your step strolling into the neonatal intensive care unit (NICU) this morning—you've been away to the mountains. Soaring peaks and towering pines in place of sepsis and cardiac arrests, you've been battling bears in place of bacteria. Mind cleared, it's back to myelomeningeoceles, intracranial hemorrhages, pre- and postmaturity, ruptured membranes and placenta previa, maternal drug abuse and infant mortality.

"God, it feels good to be home," you say.

Your role places you squarely at the nexus, your hot seat at the switch, a moment that will resolve black or white. Either all possibilities exist or none do. The neonatologist, you're responsible for the baby in the delivery room, called stat to a caesarean section when there's trouble. The population is about to ratchet up another notch—if you do your job right.

Or not, if you don't.

Right and wrong under these circumstances should be a no-brainer.

The setting is always the same. Stainless steel and tile, sterile fields and infant warmers, the surgical instruments sparkle, reflecting the large cylinders of light that beam down upon the patient. Everything is in order, all of it ready, measures to match the unfolding obstetric emergency. It's an oddly cold physical environment for such an emotionally loaded event. The father, reduced to nothing but soaring hopes and greatest fears, stands beside you, watching, waiting. Scrubbed, gowned, gloved and masked, you've never been more vulnerable to those hopes and fears. Your self-confidence has never mattered more, for doubt, a subtle hesitation or slip of the hand, snuffs out life's breath.

You're about to become "The doc who saved our baby," or "The one who didn't." And the fact is, you can't wait to prove it, make the obstetrician's day, take another rag doll and make it move, use the life stored in your fingers, make that spent baby's heart beat, make its lungs expand and fill with life-sustaining oxygen, do it in record-breaking time. All to make ecstatic moms and dads out of those people who entered the delivery room as yet unchanged by the miracle of birth, new parents who frown and puzzle and say "We didn't plan on this" when their sick babies get admitted to the NICU.

"Few parents plan on their babies coming here," you reassure them. "But aren't you glad we're here?" They never look too sure and you wonder if they have an inkling of what it's all about.

Babies and life and death, that's what.

Your work is a tremendous privilege and a terrible responsibility and you wouldn't have it any other way. But with the responsibility so grave, it's hard not to be awed by your own power.

Until you have your back against the wall, out of measures and means to employ it. Those times, you remind yourself that you and the baby are both in God's hands. Reasoning is a comfort, a salve for the baby who didn't make it, stretched out before you; reasoning is an antidote for the one who's permanently damaged no matter how fast you worked. You take refuge in those you helped, those who did make it, sat up, went to college. The whole of medicine as practiced may be gray, but the outcome in newborn medicine is often black-and-white, stark, and fraught with pitfalls.

It's hard not to take it personally.

You can't believe they pay you to assume the reins and responsibilities of the delivery room and the NICU. For the next twenty-four hours your responsibility is clear: rescue the newest arrivals from trouble; for those already present, make life advance in each isolette made of steel, glass and plastic, inanimate materials that provide critical support for the infant.

"This is Baby Boy Smith," says your colleague, signing out. He's been in charge for the last twenty-four hours. At two pounds, this baby was born eleven weeks early and has significant immature lung disease. Your colleague runs through diagnoses, speaking of RDS, PDA, IVH, a staccato clinical code documenting immature this and immature that. The usual.

That sense in you, the one most essential to the practice of medicine, kicks in: the art, and it's one of knowing who's sick and who isn't. You, all doctors, make life-and-death decisions with 50 percent of the information you'd like to have before deciding what to do next. Intuition is critical. Baby Boy Smith isn't doing well and you feel it in your well-vacationed paunch. Instinctual and automatic, it's a simple reflexive arc. Your colleague's words contain none of this despite the fact that the infant's gone from little ventilatory support yesterday to nearly maximal support today.

"He doesn't look so good," you say.

"Observe. Let the baby declare himself. Wait and watch." Can he think of one more way to say "I did nothing," or worse still, "Nothing needs to be done?" You ask questions and your colleague looks at you like you're splitting hairs. He wants to go home.

"You're not making a big enough deal out of it," you say to him, in one hundred ways other than directly, being diplomatic, then maybe not so much, as your patience is growing weary. You've been here before, this a familiar slippery slope, players the same. The faces of nurses and staff volley, your face to his, back to yours. They've all been here, too.

"I'll let you sort that out," he concedes, gives in a little, his ego—and a doctor must have a healthy one just to function in this environment—a big billowing circus tent beginning to deflate.

"The sonogram of the heart reveals a small PDA," your colleague says. "The cardiologist doubts the heart is the problem, but I think it might be."

Guesses by your colleague, but more bad ones. The cardiologist is skilled. If he doesn't think the heart's the problem, it's extremely unlikely. Something's been missed. You have twenty-three hours to show this infant a new way.

Now, you can't really complain—you do get to save a life. You're the hero here, in case you haven't figured it out. Incidentally, the reward package includes a story written, very conveniently, in second person—something you've always wanted to do.

"What does his chest X-ray show?" you ask the nurse.

"What chest X-ray?" the nurse retorts.

"The one taken after the baby was intubated and put on the ventilator," you say, thinking her question a pretty stupid one. As if such a chest film isn't always done.

"That would be which chest X-ray?" she asks again.

"There was no chest X-ray after the baby's intubation?" you say. Your own question has morphed into a deadly weapon during the asking. You've been here before—same colleague, similar baby. Baby Boy Smith's deteriorating condition is but a postcard from the past.

"Get a stat chest X-ray," you say and you're right. Initially it feels righteous, rushing to save the day.

The baby's chest X-ray shows clearly why the infant doesn't look so good. If the endotracheal tube is inserted too far (the reason why one always gets such a chest film), the baby's lungs become two balloons expanding each time the ventilator cycles a breath, pumping more air into each lung. Until they tear apart under the pressure, huge pockets of air accumulating in the baby's chest, making it impossible for his lungs to function.

"Get me chest tube setups," you say steadily, wanting to shout. But you're trained to remain cool, pursue the plan you've quickly laid out. Adrenaline pumps, that familiar sweat forms. You scrub with iodine up to your elbows, digging furiously at each nail bed.

It's something of a miracle that Baby Boy Smith is still alive, but the poison of last night's care is now dropping the infant's oxygen saturation perilously. The clock ticks, marks off increments in the remainder of this infant's life if you don't get those chest tubes in.

After local anesthesia, you cut open the chest between the fourth and fifth ribs, not unlike the bones you picked from your chicken the evening before. The baby's fragile arm is tied down, his miniature fingers wrapped round a temperature probe, fingers like worms, waving, crawling. A stream of red blood pours from the fresh cut, at least it's somewhat well oxygenated. It smarts and stings, slugs you in the gut, that you must cut this baby. This must be the gravest error, a sin of omission that cripples and tries to kill something so tiny and defenseless.

The earth's surface slows as you push the hemostat through the infant's chest wall, always surprising, the considerable force required to puncture the chest cavity of such a tiny infant, the resilience necessary to survive. The familiar "pop" of the chest wall is a gear shifting into place. The tube slides in, trapped air rushes out and, again, the earth begins turning, the violated baby's chest relaxing. You round the warmer and pop the other side of the chest wall, a similar rush of trapped air. Magic, the numbers on Baby Boy Smith's monitor stabilize. You suture the tubes into place, a cobbled bridge between good care and bad.

Over the course of your twenty-four-hour shift, you coax this tiny baby back to where he was the day before. A repeat sonogram of the baby's heart is normal. You'll sit at this baby's bedside, playing with the knobs on the ventilator, watching him wean down as the damage is reversed. Or not reversed, so much as further trauma was done to compensate for the previous damage.

In twenty-three hours, it will be time to hand Baby Boy Smith back to the man who pumped this baby's chest full of deadly pockets of air, he who might have permanently damaged this baby's lungs and significantly compromised this baby's future.

What about the others, babies who have died as a result of his incompetent care—and there have been some. Who's going to speak up for them?

This should be easy.

He's your boss; he's also your friend. "A friend may well be reckoned as the masterpiece of nature," Ralph Waldo Emerson wrote. "Be a friend and the rest will follow," added Dickens. Shakespeare: "A friend should bear his friend's infirmity." Ecclesiaticus: "A faithful friend is the medicine of life." You've always valued friendship above all. You have trouble understanding others who seemed to have no need for it. Right now, you'd like to be in their far less complicated shoes.

And it's more complicated still.

Turns out, he's the one who hired you. You'd worked together before. He wasn't so competent back then but you were both new to the field at that point. You told yourself, "He's now a seasoned veteran." "He must have improved through the years." One more way to say it, you might have believed it.

Still more complicated yet, there are only so many neonatologists and your paths are destined to continue crossing. A few years before, back when he'd been looking for work, the company you both now work for asked you for your assessment of him; you fudged a little, maybe a lot, said, "Sure, he's a fine fellow."

Because he's a good guy, right? Because you're a good guy, right? So that makes you what, a facilitator? An accomplice?

You left it at that, you couldn't really say more. So you thought, so you said, and so here you are. Working under him.

"Don't just do something, stand there," another of your physician friends loves to remind you with a smile. One of those little inside jokes that tells the whole story. The emphasis of a physician's work is upon action, especially in an emergent setting, doctors are trained to "do something." Develop a plan and get started; modify it as you go along. Emphasis on quick action turns up the heat on mistakes.

There is one caveat.

"First, do no harm." There is no more basic tenet of medical practice; all medical students learn this early. All the same, given the rapidly shifting tides of medical care, the continual need to push the limits and define new treatments, the never ending need to "do something," it's not possible to eliminate harm to patients from medical care. In highly innovative treatments such as those for AIDS and cancer, risk of harm is often high but it's something patients assume, as the alternative is deterioration and death. In reality, every treatment in a medical setting carries some risk, not unlike the risk taken driving one's car. In general, such risks are assumed and accepted.

It is widely assumed that the majority of medical mistakes are made by bad doctors. In fact, they are not. Though surveys are few in number, they show most errors occurring in the course of competent clinical care, made by consistently capable physicians. Fallibility is an inherent human characteristic. While health care is delivered through an elaborate system of checks and balances, such a human system will produce error. Physicians are acutely aware of this and, not surprisingly, given the level of their responsibility, find it an extremely difficult subject with which to grapple.

"Anyone who has ever known doctors well enough to hear medical shop talk, without reserve, knows that they are full of stories about each other's blunders and errors. . . . But no doctor dare accuse another of malpractice. He is not sure enough of his own reputation to ruin another man by it," wrote G. B. Shaw in *The Doctor's Dilemma*, most notable for its date of publication — 1911. You could swear you heard it last week.

By various rough estimates, 5 percent of physicians are incompetent. This includes those who are inexperienced and need more training, others actively alcoholic, addicted to drugs, clinically depressed, of advanced age or burnt out. While not overly abundant, information on such physicians exists. Some need rehabilitative treatment; some need additional training. Medical schools now teach students about alcoholism and drug addiction, how to spot it in oneself and others; they cover depression and the risk of burnout.

You wish your colleague fit into one of these categories. He doesn't.

This 5 percent also includes physicians whose clinical acumen is inadequate to diagnose and treat their patients' illnesses. The competent physician will make an error, but he doesn't repeat mistakes; he learns from them, delivers better care because of them. Incompetent physicians err repeatedly and in a consistent pattern, fail to learn from their mistakes, in fact, often do not realize they've made them.

The doctor as an "iatrogenic factor," making the "egregious error." Doctor as complication, as disease-maker.

Just plain bad doctors.

That is the problem you are struggling with here.

Experts in this area today describe a "norm of noncriticism," or the more inflammatory "conspiracy of silence," surrounding this issue, nothing much new under the sun on the approaching centenary of G. B. Shaw's comment.

In fact, as documented by James B. Stewart in his investigative tome, *Blind Eye,* such a conspiracy of silence, in its most malignant form, allowed a serial medical killer named Dr. Michael Swango to continue practicing medicine, killing patients for fourteen years because no one among a fairly large number of individual physicians and administrators was willing to speak out about what they had observed. Dr. Swango floated freely for years atop a whirling brew of institutional naïveté and need, old-boy-school pats on the bottom and reticence to rat on a colleague.

You almost wish your colleague was guilty of such an offense, so clearly criminal in nature. But seldom are such things so clear. Then again, what responsibility is carried by those who averted their sight while Swango continued killing? Is it not a crime, what another physician's bad care is doing to the babies under your care?

Medical students aren't taught about physician incompetence, for such would imply the system doesn't work. Students graduating from medical school represent an enormous social investment. Graduates enter a profession that, for the most part, sits above judgment; it's tricky deciding who is qualified to pass judgment on a physician. Who else has the requisite knowledge, training and experience, understands the grave responsibilities involved? Doctors' dilemmas make nearly all mortals squirm. The medical profession ends up regulating itself.

The trouble is, when he examines the mistakes of a colleague, every physician sees what Marilynn Rosenthal cites in *The Incompetent Doctor* as a "tragic version of himself." And with the increased interdependence of general practitioners, gatekeepers, and all sorts of specialists, the financial stability of a physician's practice may well depend upon referrals from the very individual undergoing scrutiny. As the bottom line becomes the top priority, these problems will only get worse.

While malpractice claims provide for a patient's recourse when "bad outcomes" occur, such cases equate these outcomes with mistakes, whether one has been made or not. Such accusations take on enormous proportions; if accused, a doctor is tried quickly by the media. The media cover the filing of the suit but aren't present when the suit is dropped or settled as a nuisance. Medical care is not a proposition with guaranteed outcomes. Some babies are going to have problems that no amount of medical care can alleviate; there is little public understanding of this.

But the murkiness in the outcome of medical practice makes a convenient place for the incompetent doctor to hide. It also provides the ready excuse for those who don't feel comfortable sitting in judgment, no matter how egregious the error, how gross the medical incompetence. In fact, that would be most physicians, most members of any group asked to critique their peers.

Eliot Freidson, in his landmark study *Profession of Medicine,* pointed out that there is a necessary reciprocation: hand-in-hand with the tremendous power and nearly absolute autonomy granted the profession of medicine comes the absolute responsibility of the profession to police itself. That is what defines it as a profession.

You, on the other hand, don't need to make expert recommendations or set policy. You just need to figure out what to do about your colleague. Truth be told, you'd rather set policy, prefer addressing the broader issue to dealing with your incompetent colleague one-on-one.

You've tried calling him on it, for the mistakes are clear at times, even to him, when you engage him in a postmortem discussion. Your scrimmage feels therapeutic, seems so clear, and then a week later, you're clambering up that slippery slope, yet again. Same mistakes, same players.

So you tell your regional medical director, the guy who supervises your part of the country for the corporation you and your colleague work for. There's a chain of command for this sort of thing and you'll follow it. You speak on the phone, spell it out. "Clinical approaches, styles of management" are pointed out to you, the centerpiece of any organization's management strategy—keep the peace, maintain the status quo. But there really isn't any style of clinical management that includes such grave insults to babies, so small and defenseless.

"Let's have lunch," he says.

Dining, discussing damaged babies. You can't quite see it.

"Sure," you say. You won't. For it's a minor problem in a big company, a temperamental fire to be stamped out.

Yeah, Yeah, Yeah, a baby's life, possibly many more.

Medicine at cost, medicine for profit.

It would be such an easy shot to blame all of this on mixing up profit and loss with right and wrong that you find it tempting. But in the end, this has little to do with money. As they say, "If your problems can be solved by money, you have very boring problems." No, this is a problem of human beings, of you and him, good care and bad. Of right and wrong, really.

This big shot then tells your colleague, your medical director, he needs to settle your "squabbles" within his own family. This comes out while you're trying, once again, to discuss another case of damage done, by him, with him. And then your colleague, your boss, your friend also starts pontificating about "clinical management styles."

Looking the other way is a management style only if malpractice is just another clinical strategy.

The baby always looks so amazing as they wheel him into court, spastic and shrunken in his high-tech wheelchair that goes forward and backward and up and down. Only problem, the child has no idea where he is at any point and isn't really going anywhere, anyway. Slobbering, malnourished, chewing on his hand, he's all jerky movements, contractions and arthrogryposes, tics, twisting and shudders, at five years of age (because that's how long it's taken to get to trial). Ka-ching, Ka-ching go the lawyers. Quite a show for the jury, whose eyes look like they're going to pop out, right down the row.

God forbid the lawyers get hold of any of these cases. Might as well settle at the limit right now—it's all over their medical records if someone knows where to look. No need to pay lawyers, a slam dunk for the damaged baby's parents.

You've told your colleague time and again, "You can fuck with me, just don't fuck with the babies."

Your philosophy of care. For you, the bottom line.

But, somehow, for him, the bottom line remains that you work "as a team, cooperate with one another. Solve our differences as a family because *team-work* is the bottom line." Yikes, you're mortified that you have some sort of role in this.

"No, *good care* is the bottom line," you say, again and again, but it's falling on incompetent and unrepentant ears.

It's not as if you haven't made mistakes yourself. You have. You will again. And, yes, this gives you plenty of pause. But not this kind of mistake, this one so like numerous other mistakes you've seen your colleague make.

The kind of mistake a medical student knows not to make.

Like a mountain range, two peaks, integrity and friendship, and in front of them, the low hills of "He helps more babies than he hurts, shouldn't he be judged on that?" You're trying to thread your way through, probing a pass between those peaks, integrity and friendship, all before the sun sets behind them. That sun's getting lower and you don't want it to set on another damaged infant.

And the whole time you keep hearing, "The hottest places in hell are saved for those who remain neutral in a time of moral crisis." What would you have done if you'd been faced with Michael Swango? The Nazis? Isn't it the same? Or is it?

You've forgotten one detail. That the ultimate responsibility does not rest with you. There are boards and bodies created to mete out justice in such instances, committees and credentialing that label and scar physicians, mangle careers, but no worse than some physicians who have mangled their patients.

You see in your mind your colleague's children no longer headed for college, his wife working as a secretary, your colleague sitting at home, depressed, moribund, finished, really.

No wonder colleagues so seldom come forward. Yes, action, that principal characteristic of most physicians—so ready to act on their patients, yet so reluctant to police their peers.

It keeps up, the ricocheting pinball machine in your head.

"Let he who is without sin cast the first stone."

"A friend in need is a friend indeed."

"The kind of mistake a medical student knows not to make."

"You can fuck with me, just don't fuck with the babies."

"Thou shalt not kill."

So, what are you going to do?

In the end, there are the babies.

Therein lies the problem.

Babies as a problem, something they should never be.

Damaged and dead babies.

God's work spoiled, not once but repeatedly.

When you reduce it to that, the only true bottom line, it begins to get easier. If you don't stand up for them, who will?

It's getting easier; you keep focusing on that damaged baby bottom line. How about this? "Friends don't allow friends to damage babies." At least not repeatedly. Those who allow it are, in fact, complicit, doing it themselves, yourself.

The next steps for you are those state boards and commissions, those agencies that reluctantly handle your complaints as gravely justified. The potential consequences for your colleague are catastrophic, but not as catastrophic as the consequences for the babies under his care.

You chose the seat at the switch, to be present when the difficult decisions about babies were being made. This is that seat, and yes, it's tougher than you imagined. You don't like to admit it but it's time to act. It is that black-and-white.

Before one more baby becomes a problem, you need to make that dreaded phone call. You pick up the phone.

No one said it would be easy.

Only that it should be.

•

Richard Beach is a board-certified neonatologist practicing in Albuquerque, New Mexico. He has also spent many years caring for AIDS patients and working in rural public health throughout Latin America.

A Merging of Head and Heart

Judith Dancoff

❧

I have a seam on my hand, a joining—the two lines that run across the palm, that are on most hands separated by millimeters of flesh, on mine are joined, as on the hand of a monkey. A simian hand is what it is called in science, a crease that marks a chromosome disorder: on the twenty-first chromosome, Down syndrome; on the eleventh, other disorders, more rare, less understood.

But I like what fortune-tellers say to the one in a million who shows up with the hand. In China they say great good fortune, at least for a boy. He is destined to be Emperor, most wealthy, very renowned; not so lucky for a girl. In Western palmistry, the predictions are equally extreme: "Because the head and heart lines are connected, the person experiences life at its most intense. This produces a single-mindedness of purpose that can yield extraordinary achievements, but also great pain." If the fate line intersects the head and heart at their place of joining, as it does on my hand—an asterisk, a small star even—the individual will be remembered for generations.

This is one prediction I find hard to believe. I have already lived half my life, and have achieved nothing extraordinary, though who can predict the future except fortune-tellers? It would certainly be a recompense, a payback, for living with this monkey hand of mine, inside this head and heart that are far too connected.

❧

A MERGING OF HEAD AND HEART

I was first diagnosed with a tumor of my pituitary gland when I was twenty-nine years old. Before that I lived most of my twenties inside a mind and body that no longer worked: sudden weight gain, depression, bouts of anger. My periods stopped, I lost all interest in sex, my pubic hair fell out, and orgasms, which had once been easy, became impossible. Though I saw a doctor every year to determine the problem, it took him seven years to come up with a diagnosis, and only because my mother read an article in *Newsweek* magazine linking birth control to lactation. Once, when I was nineteen, I lactated, and my mother never forgot that. When I told him the story, the doctor ran a blood test and then said very proudly—for they had just invented the diagnostic tool to know this—that I had a benign tumor of my pituitary, the master gland of hormones that sits just beneath the cerebral cortex. This was the cause of my problem, he said, my lack of ovulation, that had brought me to him in the first place. The tumor secreted a hormone called prolactin, responsible for nursing, but it could also stop periods. He never mentioned my sexual problems, and being a young woman in an age when all emotional or sexual difficulties were psychological, I was too ashamed to tell him. Thorough brain surgery was in order, radiation; he was excited, and I was glad too, for finally some reason might be given for all the ways my life had changed.

Mostly it was my love life that had changed. For a brief time in my late teens and early twenties, my romantic life was better than normal, so I have a clear basis for comparison. I came of age in the sexual revolution, probably my one piece of luck in all this, and I can recall telling girlfriends that my favorite thing to do in life was have sex. When a boy kissed me at the front door after a date, I would always let him in for more.

The tumor changed all that. It was not cancer, but it put me into menopause—actually worse than menopause since small amounts of hormones remain in older women's bodies, but this was not true for me. All the normal hormones shut down: estrogen, testosterone, and the numerous others that combine to make sexuality possible. I became biochemically frigid and have remained so for the majority of my adult life. I am on estrogen and other drugs today only because I sought out doctors who would put me on them. The endocrinologists who first treated me prescribed nothing. They also said nothing about sex, orgasms, libido, and I believed such questions belonged, more appropriately, in a psychologist's office. Needless to say, there were plenty of those over the years delighted to have the discussion with me.

In Eastern traditions the pituitary is considered the third eye, the window to the soul. In Western medicine it is not given such high religious status—which probably accounts for the far-too-aggressive measures taken in my treatment: the brain surgery without a CT scan and six weeks of radiation, neither of which really worked, at least not enough to restore my lost sexuality. What wasn't taken by the surgery was burned away in the radiation; still, I was not put on hormones until I asked for them myself. Imagine premature menopause, except no one tells you what's happening, or why, or offers any help, while all around you your generation is finding partners, mating, and you want to also; in fact, it is what you have lived for since childhood, since the death of your father when you were a child, except your body doesn't work.

New studies suggest that the tumor I had, a prolactinoma, is common to girls who suffer traumas with their fathers, an idea I find extraordinary, since my own father died a month before my fourth birthday. How could it be that such an event of childhood had the power to reach into my body, and thus follow me through a lifetime, on dates in the backseats of cars or inside a lover's embrace? It occurred to me recently that perhaps there is a piece of anatomy in all of us, a flap of skin that merges head and heart, that was wounded by his death, torn, the way a broken heart tears you, or how women in the olden days would die of love. I picture it as a small sheath of cells between the thalamus and cerebral cortex, a kind of eardrum. In adults it vibrates when you laugh; it keeps you healthy. You pet your cat and live longer. In children it is more sensitive; babies, untouched, die. Girls who suffer traumas with their fathers develop tumors. If so, I believe I, and people like me, have suffered the first diagnosed illness of the soul.

I first learned about my simian hand when I was seven years old. Several girlfriends were at my house after school—this was unusual; even at the age of seven I was still depressed over my father's death; it was hard for me to make friends. But today was different. A cluster of little girls in frothy dresses and petticoats ran through my living room, laughing and giggling, the sun was shining, and then one girl offered to read our fortunes, a party favor. She could say if we'd get married or not, the way her mother had taught her.

Of course we were frantic to know. It was late afternoon, and as light poured through my mother's yellow curtains, the little girl proudly showed how the lines on her hand made an "M," the way it was supposed to be. Then each of us in turn held out our hand for inspection, for the girl to trace the letter and give her approval. Like all the little girls, my own heart beat with anticipation and hope. I had heard somewhere the statistic about there being more women than men—and in my child's reasoning I assumed it meant some unlucky girls would just be passed over, maybe the unfeminine ones. I had seen a woman like that at my doctor's office, with hair on her arms that was black and thick; it was too horrible to think about.

The girl moved quickly around the circle, each hand bowed over and confirmed, like a blessing in church. Then she got to me. She looked up. There was no letter, she said flatly, no "M." I would not get married.

"Yes I will," I protested. A car drove by outside, and I tried not to cry.

"No you won't. See—the lines don't make an 'M.'"

She squeezed my palm tightly for the other girls to confirm it and showed the crease—the straight line across that said nothing. I stared with them, unable to speak, at this hand that had betrayed me.

"They have to make an 'M' for you to get married. My mother said so."

The other girls nodded assent, and clustered around me excitedly. "She's not going to get married," they whispered, looking at me with awe.

"I am too. My mother promised."

You are going to have a wonderful, loving stepfather, she would say, *and then when you get older you'll get married yourself.* She would give me this promise on nights I still cried for my father, still wanted him—his touch, the smell of his body— and as she held me on her lap, smoothing my hair, and kissing me, she would say the words: "Your husband will love you so much. Just wait. You will be very happy."

The smallest girl in the circle walked up to me, and put her finger at the center of my hand. She couldn't speak, but only peered up, her eyes wide with fear.

"Get away!" I yelled, pushing them frantically toward my front door, squeezing them out, all the ruffles and petticoats, the hot little bodies.

"Leave me alone!"

And in fact I was married briefly, two years after my operation, to a bisexual man who I sensed would not want much of me, as together we wandered the twilight of my illness, for at the time that's what it was. There were no prescriptions for estrogen or other medications, only weekly visits to a psychiatrist's office to plumb the darker reaches of my subconscious. One well-meaning therapist, I remember, had me put my uterus in a chair and talk to it. Another suggested that the pain I experienced in intercourse, the natural result of having no estrogens in my body, was, instead, a traumatic response to rape. Never mind that I had never been raped; I needed to relax. I even met with Dr. Golden, the founder of the UCLA sex clinic, who responded to my story of a pituitary tumor as though I'd just read some article in a woman's magazine about better orgasms and had cooked up the science to get an appointment with him. "Drink a glass of wine," he said. "Enjoy yourself."

The only doctor to come close to the truth was an endocrinologist in San Francisco, where I'd had my radiation treatment a few years before. He was the first person to take blood tests of my hormones, and to discover their complete absence in my body.

"Think of it like you've been castrated," he said. The summer in San Francisco was drawing to a close, and behind him a picture window looked out on the bay, the water suffused with pink light. I had just stayed up the night before writing a letter to him, trying to put into words the pain of all I had experienced, and now I was crying. He was a caring doctor. He put his arm around me as he led me back to his waiting room, but prescribed nothing. He was even a little surprised at my distress upset.

"I had a man with your illness once," he said. "He was impotent for ten years. It didn't seem to faze him at all."

∾

For most of this story I have been alone. I have not been able to share it with my best friends, not even my family. My mother, the product of a liberal Jewish upbringing, raised me in the staunch, proud belief that the power in my body was not only sacred, but also my birthright as a woman, explaining the rudiments of sex to me when I was barely five years old. "It is something you do with a person you love," she said. "It is one of the most beautiful experiences in life." And I was too ashamed to tell her the truth—that I had somehow lost that power almost as soon as I'd received it, like some precious jewel one drops in a river, and then is unable to retrieve.

There was never any question about the direction of my life, the yearning, for men, boys, love. I cannot remember a time when the feeling was not inside of me.

One of the clearest memories I have is of when I was nine years old. The boy was also nine, which makes it normal I suppose, yet at the same time all the adult components were there, the awareness of potential love, the deliciousness of the boy's body that seemed as sweet and delirious as some strange liqueur.

It happened in Marietta Hot Springs, a small, dusty mineral spa just southeast of Los Angeles. My mother, older sister and I had gone there for a week's vacation. My father had died of cancer a month before my fourth birthday, so by the time I was nine he was barely a memory. My mother, who supported my sister and me as a nursery school teacher, had little money for vacations but somehow managed to scrape the trip together with a divorced girlfriend.

I still have photographs of us from that trip: we three in our new outfits, standing by rocks, gazing at dusty roads. But what I remember most about the trip was a boy named John Block, with jet black hair and sallow skin, who went to a school close to my own, though we never saw each other again. My shorts were too tight that summer. I remember them exactly—red and white striped. I must have been growing out of them, because they cut into me, especially when we stooped together on the cool sidewalk, whispering secrets or playing games, and it got wet there, something that had never happened to me before, with a strange, new smell that made me want to be with him all the more.

That was the first real sexual experience I can remember, but it was more than sex: it was my body and soul combining to transport me to another plane. To where *my father* lived perhaps, and certainly to a place I had never experienced with my mother or sister. That was all a boyfriend was, I said to my first college roommate—with absolutely no idea of what I was saying, no cognizance of Oedipus, Electra, any of the Greeks—a father you can make love to. And I began to, as soon as I was old enough. If they were using me, I was using them too. And why not? Women's bodies were as good as men's, weren't they? Of course love was the long-term goal, but in the meantime it felt good, and if it led to something more that was great, and if it didn't, I tried not to think about it.

I look at a picture of myself from my freshman year in college—thin, tall, a fashion model really—laughing with a self-possession that seems beyond me now. I am eighteen, costumed in a small, lycra miniskirt, short bubble hair and earrings. We are on the lawn of Bennington College, at my older sister's graduation; I am three years younger, and have just broken up with my first college boyfriend. I will begin my sophomore year at UCLA in the fall.

I am in the center of the photo, my arms around my sister and stepsisters, a casualness to the tilt of my head that belies other feelings. This is the Sixties, after all, and the week before I left him, my boyfriend and I took drugs. This is really the core of the problem; the reason I can no longer be with him. Even on the lawn of Bennington College I am terrified of flashbacks, the feeling of the bad drug experience, and his face can bring it back to me whole—the fear that I will be stoned forever, that the psychosis of the drugs will never leave. I feel like I am turned inside out, like a rubber band is pulling my brain apart. Still, I look so alive in the photograph, against my sister and stepsisters who are vague and uncertain.

In retrospect, I am sure the tumor began to grow then, but silently, something no one could see. The flap of skin, perhaps, was reawakened by the drugs, the wound of my father's death retorn. A year later, I lactated — a sign there were already high levels of prolactin hormone in my brain, but of course this was misdiagnosed. The doctor at the time only said I had too much estrogen, some kind of sideways compliment to my femininity, and changed my birth control pill, which stopped the problem for a time.

I was working at the Plaza Movie Theater when it happened, down the street from UCLA. *Barefoot in the Park* was playing that week, and as Jane Fonda and Robert Redford repeated their love scenes night after night, milk would engorge my breasts. I leaned over the popcorn machine to fill bags and pour on butter, and spots of wetness would blossom on my chest. Young women had just stopped wearing bras, so there was nothing to hide the spreading wetness; when I could no longer stand it, I covered myself with a sweater and went home.

A year later, when I went off the pill for good, my periods never returned. Of course I went to doctors, but they only gave me shots and tests and told me to wait. It barely bothered me, a junior now at UCLA, studying, figuring out my life, most of all looking for love.

It has taken decades for me to figure out what happened, how all my dreams went wrong. Today, I could write chapters on each of the hormones. Take prolactin, a stress-induced hormone, that acts like a natural tranquilizer: it makes you sleepy, makes you want to nest, makes you want to be alone. Think of a nursing mother — prolactin causes the milk to flow and relaxation courses through her body. The last thing she wants is to go out and party.

Increased levels of prolactin have been found in people with chronic fatigue syndrome, Epstein-Barr, even Gulf War Syndrome, and that's also why some people on antipsychotic drugs lose interest in sex: they have too much prolactin. The drugs stop them from hallucinating but also destroy their sex lives. It has to do with the body's internal mechanism of healing, and levels are highest for people with prolactin-secreting tumors, like mine. As with any potent tranquilizer, it causes a total body shutdown: in addition to the tranquilizing effect of the prolactin, other hormones are repressed as well—estrogen, testosterone, progesterone, sometimes even adrenaline and growth hormone.

We think of medicine as a healing, a cure, but in some cases this never happens. Even after the diagnosis and the so-called treatment, the patient is left to her own devices. For years, intercourse was unbelievably painful because the tissues of my vagina had started to disintegrate, and even after I found doctors to put me on estrogen, the mystery remained, of why my libido was nonexistent, why the sensation when I did have sex or masturbate was muted and distant, a thin echo of what it once was. It's true the long-ago endocrinologist had told me to think of myself as castrated, but without the offer of a cure, maybe the truth was difficult to accept. Though I was only married for a few years, new relationships were hard to contemplate. There was too much confusion and grief every time I approached the idea of sex, and there was no help for this anywhere. "Lots of women feel so-so about sex their whole lives," I would be told by therapists, doctors, the culture at large. "Help you with your sex life? Why should I help you with your sex life? Why is that even important?"

In this state of lingering illness in which I lived, each day began pretty much the same—groggy fatigue, drag to the bathroom, turn on the news to wake up. It is true I wrote, taught English, made friends—lived, in fact, a life of health—though without all my hormones replaced, there were no peaks, no extreme feelings except fatigue, which over the years had gotten worse.

At night I would walk into my kitchen and forget why I'd come, stand for minutes eating blankly out of a bag of cereal. In the mornings I was more hopeful. I would take my newest herbal remedy and imagine a sensation in my womb, a contraction, the earliest stirrings of desire. I had the fantasy, which I could believe in for minutes at a time, that I would miraculously cure myself, my hormone levels would return to normal, and my periods would return. Then, since my ovaries were still intact, I would actually enter ten or even twenty years of womanhood—fall in love, get married, have babies. I would live my life backwards, completely out of sync with my generation, a splendid old age to match my terrible youth. Just as my sisters and friends were falling into the anxieties of menopause and beyond, I, who had lived through the worst of it, would at last be recompensed with love.

And then one evening at the college computer lab where I taught, I found the first thread, the piece of yarn I could pull to unravel the whole knot. I typed in the key words "prolactin AND sex" and waited to see what would happen. If I could just pin down the physical side of it, I reasoned, that would be a start. Naturally I wondered what would come of it, if there could actually be some answer that would reach me through the ether, and then I got a hit: an article on sex and pituitary tumors, published by an organization in Thousand Oaks, California, which called itself the Pituitary Tumor Network Association. My God, it had an 805 area code, barely ten miles from my Silver Lake apartment. I could hardly read the article without quickly flipping to the organization's Web site, its links, most of all the small star on the screen that caught my attention above everything else—"Contact Us." The next morning, with an hour or two to spare before my first class, I dialed the number.

"PTNA," a male voice answered, loud and enthusiastic.

"Hello, is this the pituitary organization?"

"Yes, ma'am. What can we do for you?"

"I need some information," I said, "about hormones, about the pituitary. I need your help."

Though I am a pituitary patient, the real suffering in my life has been my destroyed sex life. So this is what I need—not help with the tumor, but help understanding the other. Women who have total hysterectomies are in the same boat. Doctors do the operation, then leave them to figure out their ruined sex lives on their own.

I get my wish. Bob Knutzen, the cofounder of the organization, wants to meet me, and within the week we are sitting across from each other at Sol's Deli in the San Fernando Valley, eating corned beef and smoked salmon, and talking for hours.

Knutzen, who has the kind of pituitary tumor that creates giants, is a large, gregarious man with the affect of a steamroller, which he says is typical of agromegalics. Though no one has proven it, he's sure the overproduction of growth hormone stimulates the emotions of anger and aggression, just as prolactin can be associated with sadness and grief. Yes, prolactin has a calming effect, he says, but there's more to it. Think of human tears. After saline, prolactin is one of the main chemical components of tears. It is the hormone that comforts us, that bonds us, that holds us. Perhaps women, who cry more easily than men, do so because they have more of the hormone.

When he talks about his subject, his eyes light on fire, the pickle in his hand shaking as he makes this point or that. Bob is not a small man; maybe his hands are a little large, his forehead, but otherwise he looks entirely normal, as I know I must look to him. Our diseases are only visible on the inside.

After undergoing operations at two Los Angeles hospitals, Bob began the organization, with his doctor on the board of directors. Like me, he is sexually dysfunctional, and has other problems too. Top doctors and scientists around the world are now on PTNA's board of directors, and still no one gets it, he says, his face reddening. They treat you for the tumor, fine, but then they leave you hanging. How are you supposed to live your life?

"So here's the deal, Judy," he says. I have called myself Judith since the age of thirteen, since my mother married my stepfather, but coming from Bob, Judy sounds good. He stubs his index finger into the table to make his point. "How would you like a brand-new computer in exchange for doing PR?"

Of course I answer yes.

"We've got to get this information out!" he stresses, stuffing half a corned beef sandwich into his mouth.

And more than just getting a computer, I will learn about hormones, about the pituitary, maybe even figure out how to make my body work. An hour before, while waiting for him at Sol's Deli, I'd had brief fantasies that we would meet and fall in love, two wounded beings coming together for commiseration and love. This is typical of me—to fantasize love in any situation—but Bob has been married for decades and has a grown family. Besides, his interest is not personal. He believes that medical science will save him, if only he can encourage enough doctors to invent the right medicines.

At the same time, Bob is lucky. When agromegaly goes uncontrolled, the feet, hands and jaw become huge, the spine shoots up a foot or two; the person can become eight feet tall. Some agromegalics go undiagnosed for decades because their family physicians are too ignorant to run a blood test; by the time they are circus giants, little can be done. It is not true that people with great physical deformities learn to adapt well. Many women with mastectomies get counseling, paid for by their insurance; not so for pituitary patients. And yet pituitary tumors are unbelievably common, Bob says. In random autopsies, scientists have found pituitary tumors in 25 percent of the population.

Driving home that day, I think again of the tears and prolactin and it makes sense—how sad I was when the illness first began, how confused. The women's movement was in full swing, I wore work boots and went on marches. When I first went to my doctor, years before his diagnosis, he puzzled a moment or two over the fact that my periods had stopped and shrugged. "Come back in six months," he said. Maybe my periods would return by then. "And if not, well, I guess you're not the kind of woman to want children anyway," he concluded, looking over my clothes and lack of makeup, the straightforward tilt of my jaw. At the time he was the top endocrinologist at Kaiser Permanente, Los Angeles. I had seen him the year before when I first told him about the lactation, but he paid no attention, and would not for many years, until my mother read the *Newsweek* article. In the darker regions of my soul, maybe I believed what he said was partly true. At the age of twenty-three, I was still trying to reason out why people I loved might reject me; how I could bring that on, so much pain and heartache. I can remember hating the feeling in my body, the desire for sex and love, and actually wishing it away.

Some scientists now believe that the hypothalamic/pituitary/adrenal axis is the neurobiological center of human emotion; that emotions are not just strange humors wafting through our veins, but actual, physical realities that inhabit our bodies.

There is a new field at colleges nowadays called Consciousness Studies, which combines philosophers, psychologists, biologists, neurologists—all looking into this question of head and heart, mind and body, trying to find the center of it for the first time. And it may indeed be located in a sheath of skin between our thalamus and cerebral cortex. But consciousness is more than simple anatomy, they say. It is the thing that makes the color red *red*, the sound of middle C, the joy of orgasm. It is an irreducible truth of the universe, like gravity or time, that only enters our bodies while we are alive. In yoga, it is the light that enters your soul through your third eye, your pituitary.

And if they had located this center of consciousness in me when I was twenty-three, what would they have found? The torn flap of skin, the sheath between my thalamus and cerebral cortex, soothed by prolactin hormone, upset by the drug trip, a faithless lover, still pained by my father's death?

Bob and I stand in the parking lot a few extra minutes, exchanging notes and phone numbers. He gives me the title of a book about sex and hormones, which will go a long distance toward unraveling my confusion; I give him names of people to call for marketing and publicity. When I finally pull onto the Ventura Freeway, I feel a small window open up inside of me. How is it that a life can seem to be going in one direction so completely, and end up so entirely reversed? It will be a long time before I fully understand, but I have taken the first step.

•

Judith Dancoff *lives in Los Angeles, surrounded by several cats and many wonderful friends. Her fiction and essays have appeared in* Other Voices, *the* Alaska Quarterly Review, Mademoiselle, *and* L.A. Weekly. *She is also a documentary filmmaker; her movies have screened at the Whitney Museum and the National Museum of Women in the Arts.*

Interesting Case

Do Not Discard

Natalie Smith Parra

∾

My cancer started five and a half years ago with a barely noticed mass on a routine chest X-ray. I'm in Target buying paper towels and bathroom hooks when the nurse pages me. I leave my shopping cart near the check stand and go outside to call her from a pay phone.

"There's a mass on your left lung," she says. "Can you come in for a CT scan this afternoon? Anytime before 5:30?"

"Yes, yes," I tell her, "of course." I don't really know what a mass on the lung means, exactly how a CT scan works, or what it will show.

The first of my many CT scans takes place in a windowless room of the hospital basement. I lie on the table while a doctor injects dye into the bulging vein in the crook of my arm. Above my head to the left, the word Siemens is inscribed in black on a silver metal plate attached to the machine. I think of Judy Chicago's "Holocaust Project," and I see the gaunt shaved-head slave laborers shuffle into the Siemens factory. The thought occurs to me to jump up, to demand a different machine, a boycott of Siemens, but I'm entering a parallel world now, one in which I will learn to be quiet. I will learn to comply, to submit. I will learn to live outside the tumultuous world as if watching a windstorm from the inside of a car. I haven't yet crossed the border into this new world, but I am definitely in the border region.

Afterward the radiologist comes out from behind an enclosure. His eyes are puffy and brown, his hair gunmetal gray. He speaks to me softly, his eyes trained on his shoe.

"What are you here for?" he asks.

"I'm not sure," I say, swinging my legs off the table. "Something about something on my lung."

He nods. As I leave he wishes me good luck. I smile and shrug. I am thirty-eight years old. I still feel the invincibility of my youth. I'm not yet too worried about this mass, which I figure will be cleared up with some kind of pill.

The next time the nurse calls me I am at home after work, exhausted after teaching five periods of high school English. I am staring at last night's dirty dinner dishes and wondering why neither my son nor daughter has washed them after school.

"Natalie," she says, "there's definitely a mass there. It looks pretty small, about two square centimeters."

"That's good," I say. When she doesn't answer quickly enough I ask, "Isn't it?" I want to know what it could be, the range of possibility. "Is it cancer?"

"It could be," her voice is cautious, "but it could be something else, some kind of infection. There are some enlarged lymph nodes in the area." My ignorance of cancer is so thorough that I think enlarged lymph nodes in the area are a good thing. Don't you get enlarged lymph nodes when you have a sore throat? A cold? In my new world, a whole other body of knowledge with its own vocabulary is necessary. The nurse makes an appointment for me with the thoracic surgeon on Thursday.

In the surgeon's waiting room, my mother sits under the window, her black bag clutched to her chest, ankles crossed. She will be my constant shadow now, she tells me. Whenever I go to an appointment, she will go too. Despite her maternal posturing, she seems diminished, shrunken against that sea-green wall.

First a tall young resident with an Eastern European accent introduces himself. He is wearing black felt clogs and green scrubs. He asks a lot of questions, jots down my answers. Then the door pushes open and silence descends on the room as the surgeon enters; he has thin gray hair that hangs over the collar of his white coat, his gray beard could use a trim. He has watery eyes and gold-rimmed glasses push down on his nose. He flips his calendar open to December. "How will the 12th be?" he asks.

"Wait, wait," I hold up my hand. "Aren't we here to talk about options? Tests? Biopsies? Or something? The nurse told me that you can take a sputum sample with a bronchoscope. How about that?"

Dr. Wagoner shakes his head. "Bronchoscopies are for people I don't want to operate on. You have a small mass; we'll remove it. Simple."

"Excuse me, Doctor," my diffident, polite mother speaks. "If this were your daughter, would you recommend going outside the HMO if we could get the operation done a month earlier? Would that give her a better chance?" She twists the straps of her bag. For the first time my mother looks like a very old woman.

The surgeon presses his lips together, shakes his head. "What are you saying?" His gaze falls on my mother, who shrinks deeper into her chair. "Are you suggesting that I would risk your daughter's life? If that's what you think, maybe you should try another surgeon. Here. I'll give you a referral." He reaches for his pocket. I jump off the table, sliding my feet into backless shoes.

"Yeah. Good idea. Go ahead; write it," I say. The resident jerks his head up. Wagoner and I lock eyes for a moment. I glance at my mother, who is squeezing a wad of tissue in one hand.

"No, no, no," my mother says. "Please, Natalie. Doctor, we want you to do the operation. We've heard you are a good surgeon." I glare at my mother, then start to speak, but I can't. My mouth is filled with sand.

A small, satisfied smile crosses Wagoner's face. My mother wipes her nose. "Good, okay then," he says. "Would it make you feel better if we move it up a week? Say, to December 5th?" He turns and leaves the room.

The resident explains the surgery to me. Three weeks from now they will perform a thoracotomy, where they open the thorax by cutting through the rib cage. Pneumonectomy is the removal of the lung, but what will happen once my chest is opened will depend on what the surgeon sees inside. "Now," the residents says, "I'll get you set up for your pre-op blood work." I can hear my ribs crack, dry twigs breaking.

The operation is supposed to last four or five hours, so when my family — husband, mother, two oldest kids, sister, ex-husband — see Wagoner step out of the elevator with a tie hanging down the inside of a clean white coat, his hair wet and combed, they think I'm dead. It has only been two hours, maybe a little less. They think that with surgery, you either survive it or die. Wagoner motions for them to sit in an alcove in the corner of the waiting room. They leave their take-out Chinese food picnic on top of outdated copies of worn magazines, chow mein noodles dripping down the sides of white cardboard cartons.

Wagoner tells them that it is cancer and that it's spread to lymph nodes all over my chest. Taking out the lung wouldn't have helped so he just closed me back up. He says he'll refer me to an oncologist; maybe there's some chemotherapy for me, but he doubts it. It's much worse than he thought. He tells them he is going home; he'll be back to talk to me in the morning; in the meantime, he suggests that my family not discuss the situation with me.

My son Jonathon remembers watching the elevator come and go, filled with medical staff, walk-in patients and visitors, arms loaded with balloon bouquets, flowers, stuffed animals. "It wasn't even a private thing," he said.

Later my mother remembers, "Dr. Wagoner said, 'I'm very sorry.'"

"He did?" I ask. "It doesn't sound like him."

She tilts her head, wondering. "Well, yes, wouldn't he say something like that after he tells you your daughter is going to die?"

I wake up in the recovery room, my bed the last in a row of seven or eight. At first the lights are too bright for me to open my eyes. When I am able, I look down the row and feel some relief that the stiff white sheets are pulled only to the patients' chins, so I know I'm not in the morgue. My body is a dry leaf, parched, and I beg for water. A young nurse with a thick dark ponytail and clear skin feeds me ice chips against Wagoner's orders. We talk about our kids. She has two. She says that without her union, Wagoner would have had her fired. "He's an asshole," she says, and I smile.

"I know," I say. "I hate him."

My head is heavy and thick with morphine, and my lips feel as if they've been pulled around a rubber ball. My eyes strain to focus and finally land on the surgeon sitting next to my mother on a hard chair against the wall. My mother's arms are crossed and her lips are pressed tight. Her face betrays her exhaustion. The doctor and my mother aren't talking. Why is he here in the middle of the night? I want to know. But it's not night anymore. It's my first morning in the parallel world. On the hospital tray, next to a mustard-colored pitcher of water, lies a brochure about hospice care—a fifty-something woman with stylish salt-and-pepper hair smiles and gazes up into a younger man's face, her son's, most likely. They are both happy with their decision about end-of-life care. When Wagoner sees me trying to focus on the brochure, he ignores me and talks to my mother. "She could go to hospice for pain," he says. My mother's eyes meet mine.

"I didn't have any pain until this operation," I say. He lets out a short laugh.

I draw my veil of denial tight around me. I won't accept his prognosis. I can't. I have a four-year-old child to raise, eleventh-grade students to teach, a world to change. I am supposed to die an old woman, happy, sitting in front of my window watching a revolution in the streets.

The HMO says wait until after the holidays to start chemotherapy. So I do.

∾

On Christmas Eve, cold and cheerless and gray, my mother, my sister and I drive across town to an appointment with Dr. Denise Manning at a large university cancer center. She is their expert on lung cancer and cancers of unknown origin. She will act as a second opinion in terms of what kind of chemotherapy the HMO should be giving me and in which doses. The cancer center has free valet parking and an art deco interior with flagstone walkways; its television advertising is directed at an upscale clientele. But despite the wreaths and Santa faces hanging on the walls and doors, the cancer center is a quiet and grim place on Christmas Eve.

In one of the billing cubicles a polyester-pant-suited woman with orange lipstick and a beehive hairdo clicks away at a computer. No doubt her mind is filled with all the things that need to be done: her unwrapped Christmas presents, the turkey waiting to be stuffed and roasted. She dispenses with niceties. No Merry Christmas, good afternoon, how are you feeling. She cuts to the chase. "How will you be paying today?"

"Check," I say. I write the check for five hundred dollars and slide it across the desk, letting my fingers rest on it for just a second, long enough to make her look up, then I say, "Where do I go now?"

"Sit there. Someone will call you."

Across the big desk from us, Dr. Manning flips through my file, pauses where something interests her and then flips some more.

My sister pulls a bouquet of Tootsie Pops, orange, purple, red, brown, from her bag and offers one to the doctor.

"Oh, yeah, thanks," Dr. Manning says, reaching across the desk. "Sugar is my weakness." She chooses the red one, unwraps it and swirls it around inside her mouth as she talks. She wields the red Tootsie Pop like a pointer. "Well," she says, aiming it at me now. "Your cancer is Stage Three."

I nod.

She catches my eyes with her own. "B. Stage Three B," she says with authority.

"I know," I say, but I'm lying so I can get home and rest. The truth is I have no idea that my cancer is Stage Three B, never operable, instead of Three A, which often is. So far, no one has bothered to explain it to me. I am too tired and hopelessly uninformed to formulate the question that seems so simple now: Why Three B instead of Three A?

Months later I learn that Stage Three is divided into A and B. In A, the lymph nodes on the same side as the tumor are involved. This is considered operable, depending, as I would soon learn, on the skill level and attitude of the attending surgeon.

Stage Three B is inoperable. The cancer has spread to the lymph nodes on the opposite side of the chest. The difference between Three A and Three B may be determined at diagnosis by a mediastinoscopy, a sample of lymph node tissue on both sides of the trachea—the test Wagoner didn't bother with, instead sawing me open, taking a disgusted look inside, and stapling me back together. Dr. Manning now labels me a Stage Three B to fit the medical model that Wagoner has constructed. Stage Three B becomes an established fact of my medical diagnosis, completely without a biologic sample.

Dr. Manning recommends chemotherapy, Taxol and carbo platin, and my lawyer sister pops a chocolate sucker into her mouth. "Listen, I've been thinking," she says, and points her Tootsie Pop at the doctor. "I say if that's the recommended amount, we double it. The more the better, the way I see it. Let's be aggressive here."

Dr. Manning's eyes grow wide, and her cheeks suck in to hold the red Tootsie Pop in place. "I don't want to kill your sister," she says and smiles. But she never suggests any further tests or a need for further data.

The chemo nurse rubs her thumb over the back of my hand. "You have good veins," she says. Jeanne is short and chubby with a pinkish face and blond hair wisping around her neck. My mother stands at the door and watches the nurse hang the first slick bag: Taxol, made from the bark of the Pacific yew tree.

Later in the afternoon my mother browses the newspaper. I lean back in my reclining chair, tethered to an IV pole by a plastic tube now dripping carbo platin into the crook of my arm. I'm still drowsy and thick-tongued from the Benadryl they gave me with the Taxol to prevent allergic shock. Outside it rains without stopping. The month since my diagnosis has been the coldest month ever. Some days the water comes down in ropes, sometimes in cascading lead sheets. Rubber trashcans wash down the steep hills near downtown. The sky stays dead and heavy and gray, the same gray as the ocean, the gray of the streets.

The oncologist comes in wearing her white coat with the name patch and the ink stains on the pocket. She presses my thick file chart to her chest.

"How many people with this disease have you cured?" I ask. The doctor looks down, lets out breath. Her knuckles whiten on the edges of the folder. "No one," she says.

When she sets my file on a counter I see a hexagonal yellow sticker emblazoned with black letters: Interesting Case: Do Not Discard.

I shouldn't have asked. I already know the answer. I've known it for a month now, since I woke up in the greenish-gray glow of hospital lights.

After eighteen weeks of chemotherapy I start radiation treatments. You can receive up to 5,000 rads of radiation to the chest before things start to fall apart. Tissue doesn't hold together well and there is the danger of bleeding to death during surgery, so halfway through my eight-week course of radiation, I call Wagoner.

"How are you?" he asks.

"Alive," I say. "I think the chemo is working. I'm feeling good, and I want an appointment with you to reassess my potential for surgery." By now I know that without an operation I have between a 1 and 5 percent chance of living out the year.

I hear him let out breath on the other end of the phone. He agrees to see me. Call the receptionist to make an appointment, he says.

On Friday morning Wagoner is surprised by my good health. He barks at the nurse to order an emergent CT scan and tells me to come back on Monday afternoon to review the results with him. I go home full of hope. I even think that I may have it all wrong about Wagoner. Maybe I misunderstood him.

"He didn't seem so bad today," I tell my family. My mother and my sister shoot each other a look that I pretend not to see. I call my friends to tell them the good news.

On Monday my mother, sister and I cram into the tiny examining room. I lie on the table anxious and excited. I breathe in, count the seconds, breathe out, do it again, the way they showed me in the visualization and relaxation classes. We're waiting too long, I think. The news must be bad, otherwise wouldn't he rush in, all smiles? When he finally pushes through the door his expression is neutral.

"I have bad news," he says. "There's been no change. An operation is out of the question."

"But you said I'd be dead by now, and I'm fine."

"I don't know how to explain that."

"What about the chemo? Are you saying it's had no effect?"

"Completely ineffective."

"Has the cancer spread? Is it any bigger?"

"No, no, I really can't say that it's any bigger." Later I find out there's no way to determine whether tumor tissue is dead or alive without a biopsy. He could have ordered a biopsy but he didn't.

I leave the examining room and start down the long hall toward the exit. A rush of tears chokes me. A receptionist sees me and turns away.

"I'm sorry." I hear Wagoner's voice and turn around. He is standing in the hall flanked by my sister and mother.

"It's not your fault," I whimper, and for the first time since December, I think that maybe he has done all that he can.

"You can stay in my office if you want, until you feel better."

When will I feel better? When my lungs fill quietly with fluid and I die in my sleep, as another doctor recently told me? Or maybe, if I sit in his office, I'll feel better in just a few minutes about dying. I almost smile. I shake my head. No, it's not necessary. I'm not worried about any embarrassment I might feel making my way through his crowded waiting room crying like a small child. I keep walking, threading my way around chairs filled with patients watching me with quizzical and sympathetic eyes. My sister and my mother follow a short distance behind me, stunned and silent, into the elevator and out of the cool clinic into the bright summer sun, the heat, the horns bleating, the fumes. All those people and me. I feel as though a clear cylinder has been dropped over me, separating me, finally and fully, from the world I know.

This is what I remember of the next three days: The two oldest of my three children are waiting when I get home. When they realize what is happening they run out of the room in tears. I sit, elbows propped on the rough pine table, reviewing insurance forms. I take a tranquilizer and sleep. Death is certain now. A few months ago I had contacted Elaine Beech, the coordinator of a retreat for cancer patients. Now she calls to see if I plan to attend. I wrap the black phone cord around my finger and tell her I can't decide right now. I don't know when I'll be able to tell her. I take more Ativan and sleep. I leave three messages on Wagoner's voice mail before I finally catch him at his desk.

"I need to know exactly why surgery can't work for me," I say.

A long, frustrated exhalation.

"Has the cancer spread too far or is it because of the tumor's proximity to my aorta?"

"What do you want me to do?" His voice is barely restrained anger. "Cut you open and staple you back up like I did before?"

"No, no, I just want to understand. I'm sorry. What do you think my chances are now of surviving a year?"

"Less than 1 percent. Is that what you wanted to hear?" he says.

"Okay, thank you. Good-bye."

"Okay, good-bye."

Elaine Beech calls again. I order my kids to tell her I'm not home. Once I pick up the phone, not thinking, and it's her.

"Listen," she says. "I don't want you to take that surgical opinion as a death sentence."

"Uh, okay. Whatever."

"I have the phone number of a very good lung surgeon. Maybe you should make an appointment."

"Okay. Thank you."

I take more Ativan and go back to sleep. She calls the next morning and I shake my head.

"Tell her I'm not here," I motion to my son.

The only tolerable position is stoned on Ativan, curled into a fetal position in a dark room with my face buried in a cool pillow. No sight, no sound, no light. I'm like an infant that twists and twitches itself into the birth position, readying itself for life, except that I am preparing for death.

Now that all hope is gone, I am not accepting death well. There is nothing left to rage against, nothing to fight. My own body has betrayed me, and it will win. I feel none of the peace associated with the so-called other side. There is just me, then not me, the world without me in it. I want to buy my four-year-old daughter a winter coat for every year I won't be with her, but that won't do. She will need so much more.

Elaine Beech calls again. I tell her I'm sick of doctors poking me and looking at me like I'm already dead. I have run out of energy for doctors.

"Please, Natalie," she implores. "What can one more appointment hurt?" I think about her question. I would have to uncurl myself, leave my bedroom and go out into the light. I would have to make polite conversation with a receptionist and a nurse.

"No," I say. "I appreciate your concern, but I don't think I can do it."

The next day she calls three times before she reaches me.

My mother says, "We might as well go. That way, if he says no too, we'll know we did all we could."

At another university medical center the doctor finally orders my first mediastinoscopy—a biopsy of the lymph nodes of the trachea. A week after the

procedure, I wait for results. If the lymph nodes on the left are the only positive ones, I will be able to have surgery. My chances of surviving until the end
of the year will then jump from less than 5 percent to somewhere around 35
percent. It's my best hope, my last real chance. If the cancer has spread to the
opposite nodes, surgery is not an option. A mediastinoscopy is the test
Wagoner should have done first. Instead, it has taken from early December
until now, late July, for me to have this test.

The new surgeon, Dr. Cameron, is unhappy with the CT films I've
brought from the HMO. He clucks his tongue, "They didn't even use
contrast." In addition to a suitable CT scan, Cameron also orders an MRI of
the brain, a bone scan and a positron-emission tomography (PET) scan, a
newer technology the HMO doesn't even use yet, to rule out distant metastasis. I have passed all the tests. The mediastinoscopy will determine if
surgery is appropriate.

I drive west on the way to my youngest daughter Sasha's swimming lesson.
The amber light of summer casts shadows on sidewalks, and the air begins to
cool from another scorching day. In the distance the sky glows gold and pink.
I watch pigeons, puffs in shades of gray and white, burst from an abandoned
brick building and fly in a perfect arc toward the sunset. How could these
birds, that scrape flattened crumbs of bread off the asphalt of the school playground and bathe in the fetid water of the city's gutters, choreograph a flight
so fragile, so perfect? For an instant I believe anything is possible. I sit on a
wood bench next to the pool and run my finger over its scarred surface, years
of initials and proclamations of love and profanities scraped into the old
wood. Sasha is the best swimmer in her class of four-year-olds. She is kicking
up sparkling shards of water, oblivious to my tortured waiting. I step outside
the gate to check my messages. Dr. Cameron's voice is excited. He has good
news. We can schedule the surgery. I cry as my fingers fumble to dial his
number on the cell phone.

"Oh good. It's you," his secretary says. "He wants to talk to you."

"The pathology report shows no evidence of disease in any of your lymph nodes," he says, "not even on the left side. What Wagoner saw on the films was totally dead tissue." As an afterthought Cameron says, "By the way, the HMO has already admitted they are incapable of performing the operation, so they have to pay for it."

The HMO pays for lots of procedures at other medical centers: bone marrow, liver, heart and lung transplants.

The trick, though, is that the HMO surgeon must refer the patient and authorize the payment. I leave messages with everyone I can think of: heads of departments, membership services, six or seven a day on Wagoner's voice mail. My oncologist is out of town.

The day before my scheduled surgery, Liliana, an old friend and a longtime clerical worker at the HMO, and I meet outside her building on her lunch break, and together we walk in silence the few blocks to the clinic building. We pass the unmarked side entrance to the basement where the CT scan machines are kept, and stop in front of a vase of orange chrysanthemums on the stone steps of the main hospital building. Liliana had introduced me to David Trang's mother, who put the flowers there. She makes this pilgrimage every day in memory of her son, who died in that building of leukemia at ten, diagnosed after a year of various antibiotic therapies failed to cure his stomach pains and general malaise—too late for a life-saving bone marrow transplant. I've seen her leaflet in front of the HMO. She writes about the mistreatment of her son and the doctor who tried to insert an adult-sized catheter in David's tiny penis, then laughed at her when she complained about his pain. "You better get used to that. He has leukemia now," he said.

Stepping out of the elevator we hear a distant voice and follow it to Liz, a surgery department secretary speaking into a headset and sipping Diet Coke. Liliana and Liz acknowledge each other with a nod.

"I need to see Dr. Wagoner," I say.

Liz looks confused. "Do you have an appointment?"

"No, but my surgery is scheduled for tomorrow, and he should have left me an authorization form."

"Well, he's not here, and he didn't leave anything with me." She raises an eyebrow and slurps the rest of her Diet Coke. "I don't know how to help you, ma'am." She turns away.

"Come on, Liz," Liliana says. The tone of her voice goes from the easy banter of coworkers to impatient, irritated. "Who's the chief of surgery here? Let's locate him, okay?"

Liz disappears for a couple of minutes and then returns. "Dr. Pizaro's on a phone conference. He says he'll come out to see you in a few minutes." We sit in the orange plastic chairs and thumb through wrinkled copies of *Business Week* and *Golf Digest*.

We wait another ten minutes for Dr. Pizaro, chief of surgery, to finish his telephone conference, but when he emerges from an office dressed in street clothes and carrying a briefcase he hurries by us to the elevator.

"Uh, excuse me." Liliana says and motions to me. I step in front of him and plead my case.

Dr. Pizaro looks away, checks his watch and looks back. The skin under his eyes looks smudged. "There's nothing I can do about that. It's a case I know nothing about."

"Can't you get in touch with Wagoner?" I ask "Can't you call Dr. Cameron? Can you even look in my chart so you will know something about my case?"

"I'm in a hurry now. I'm on my way to a meeting." He glances at his watch again and lifts his briefcase as proof. "Maybe if you call me tomorrow." He tries to thread his way past us, but we stay with him. He can't move without pushing one of us out of the way.

Liliana takes a step closer to Dr. Pizaro. "You're the chief of surgery." She points an accusing finger. "You didn't get that title for nothing and we're not leaving until you do something. What happened to all that bullshit about patient care? We're not leaving. We'll stand here until you give us the form or until security drags us away, and that won't look very good, will it? And even if that does happen, we'll be back, and we'll bring friends, lots of friends."

Dr. Pizaro sighs and sets his briefcase on a counter. He pulls his wallet from his back pocket and thumbs for a card. "Here," he hands it to me. "Have your surgeon page me, and if the story makes sense, I'll approve it."

"Thanks," I take the card and wipe at my tears with the back of my hand.

"Well," Liliana says, smiling. "I'd better get back to work, so I'm not late from lunch."

My surgery is scheduled for six A.M. At that early hour, before the heat of July begins to broil the city, Dr. Cameron will open my chest and remove my whole left lung. Then he will gently slice my pericardium, the thin membrane under which lies my beating heart, and scrape away any tumor that has attached itself to my aorta. I'm not a bit nervous. I feel a vague anticipation like I feel when I have to get to the airport.

When I arrive at the hospital the receptionist tells me that the HMO hasn't notified them of the approval to pay. Other patients look up and shake their heads. A mother holds and rocks her small daughter, strokes her hair, kisses the top of her head. The girl will have a kidney transplant today. An old couple holds hands. Infuriated, I punch Wagoner's number on the pay phone hanging next to the waiting room door. Of course there is no answer. I call back several times leaving a series of messages. "I'm standing here waiting to go into the OR," I say. "Now you're holding up the whole surgery schedule. I hope you're happy." The receptionist smiles and shakes her head.

"Will you call Dr. Cameron?" I ask. "Maybe he's heard something."

A few minutes later she summons me to her desk. "He wants me to send you in," she says. She doesn't say whether the HMO has approved the payment or not. I have the operation without knowing.

The next morning Dr. Cameron pulls a chair to the side of my bed. "The operation was a success," he says. We sit and smile at each other for a few minutes, both shaking our heads in disbelief. He tells me that he removed my left lung, and when he started to work on the tumor around the aorta it was already hard and dead, like dry clay.

"I touched it with a scalpel," he says, "and it fell right off. Dead tissue."

"Why did Wagoner tell me nothing had changed?" I ask.

"He just looked at the CT films, which can show live or dead tissue. That's why, in cases like this, you definitely need a biologic sample. You had an excellent, if not complete, response to the chemotherapy."

It isn't a cure, he reminds me. Cancer is tricky, but he's optimistic. He will watch me closely for the next five years. Five years, five years, five years — like an incantation. The words dance in my head.

•

Natalie Smith Parra is a native of Los Angeles, where she is at work on a book of creative nonfiction. She was recently awarded writing residencies at Hedgebrook and Mesa Refuge and a grant from the Money for Women/Barbara Deming Memorial Fund.

Hypoplastic Heart

Ron Grant

∾

One afternoon some years ago, I drove a baby to the morgue in my Jeep. Nathan Spann was three weeks old when he succumbed to hypoplastic left heart syndrome, a rare congenital disorder in which the left heart ventricle — the chamber responsible for pumping oxygenated blood from the lungs into the aorta and then out to the body — is underdeveloped and fails. At the time of the diagnosis, the three-step corrective procedure used extensively today was in its infancy, leaving Stefan and Roni — a doctor and nurse — with only two viable options: A heart transplant or a natural death in the comfort of his home.

"Will you come to the house when Nathan passes away?"

Stefan and Roni posed their terrifying question the day after learning their son's bleak prognosis. Nathan had just turned a week old, and the visit to my office that day should have been one of weight and height measurements and discussions of feeding habits and developmental milestones. Instead, we sat talking bluntly about the potential complications of open-heart surgery, insurance costs related to the length of the hospital stay, and the possibility of his having to be on immunosuppressive medications for life.

It was the spring of 1994 and the practice of medicine was in the midst of a face-lift. Having practiced pediatrics for a couple of years, I was already witnessing health maintenance organizations shifting patient control from the practitioner to the administrator and restricting the number of laboratory tests we could order, the antibiotics we could choose, and the amount of time our patients could remain in the hospital. Newborn education, normally initiated when mothers were still in their obstetrical rooms and their babies in the nursery, was now being completed in the physician's office.

Office time in those first few visits was spent discussing feeding habits and neonatal emergencies as well as answering parenting questions. How many hours between feeds, what are the pros and cons of nursing, and what kind of formula do four out of five doctors recommend? What rectal temperature constitutes a fever and whom do we call at three in the morning if the infant is sick? Which brand of car seat do we buy and where in the vehicle is the safest place to locate it?

"Will you come to the house when Nathan passes away?"

The room filled with silence as I stared across my desk, first at the Spanns, and then up at my diplomas that were hanging on the wall behind them. This couple weren't just parents of a patient, but good friends. Three years before, sitting in the same chairs, they had picked me as their pediatrician, and from that moment on the relationship had blossomed. I occasionally ran into Stefan at the medical center and Roni often joined me at Gymboree (a gymnastics-like play center for babies and toddlers) as well as Children's Park, where our two-year-olds played together in the sand and swings with children of other health-care professionals.

Roni and I came from similar backgrounds—we were both firstborn child of liberal Jewish parents—and our friendship was cultivated in the office and on the playground where we often had intense philosophical discussions. No topic was off-limits. We talked about women's rights, religious mantras, and politics. We talked about interfaith marriage, capital punishment, gun control, and how our liberal leanings were often at odds with others in our profession. We talked about euthanasia, both of us agreeing that the quality of life takes precedence over one wrought with long-term pain and suffering. And of course, we talked on and on about our two-year-olds. Zachary, her firstborn, was a bright and rambunctious child who knew his alphabet forward and backward, could understand short readers, and loved to squeeze the rubber gloves I blew into balloons between his fingers, squealing with delight when they exploded. He especially loved to wiggle out of my grasp whenever I tried to hold him in my lap and look in his ears.

As I contemplated the Spanns' painful question, I thought back to some of the specifics of our conversations: our dismay at the country's conservative political turn, our desire to be at an arm's length from our loving, but over-protective, parents, and the religious choices our spouses had made. My wife Jennifer had converted to Judaism before our marriage, but Stefan, not being religious, had not, and we discussed how those differences in our respective relationships had affected our practice of religion in the home. We even talked about circumcision—a *bris* being one of the most traditional of Jewish ceremonies—and I had performed Zachary's, because Stefan, not Roni, had requested it.

I had also performed a circumcision on Nathan the day after his birth— the only time I saw him before his death. During the week I had talked to Roni on the phone several times: she was excited to have another newborn boy in the house, a baby that she called a Zachary clone. Not only did they look alike, they had similar mannerisms: sleeping with a tiny hand tucked underneath their belly, and pursing their lower lip in a downward curl when they cried.

But unlike his brother at that age, Nathan couldn't seem to satiate. At first, Roni assumed that Nathan's excessive hunger was simply due to his genetic makeup and she tried to keep up with his tremendous demand by feeding him more often. But then his feeding time began to grow long, and as the intervals between them disappeared, she became concerned, phoning the clinic when his face turned dusky blue while she was nursing him.

The pediatrician on call wanted to examine Nathan immediately. "Newborns can get blue around the lips if they choke on their milk," he said. "It's probably nothing to worry about, but we should check him out. Meet me at the ER in twenty minutes."

Three hours later, in the same exam room in which Stefan had once sutured an eight-year-old's facial laceration, an echocardiogram of Nathan's chest revealed a barely functioning left ventricle, and a few minutes later, a young-looking surgical resident with stubble on his chin walked into the room. He examined Nathan briefly and immediately began talking heart transplant. He was wearing bloodstained, oversized scrubs and leaned casually against the wall as he talked about low cardiac output, poor end-organ perfusion, and the new and exciting transplant work that he and his colleagues were currently performing.

"We need some time to digest this," Stefan finally interjected. "I'm going to make some phone calls, talk to a few colleagues, check a couple of articles. But for the moment, we're taking Nathan home. Roni and I need some time to discuss our options."

"There are no options," the resident replied. "It's either a heart transplant or the baby dies. It's that simple. And the sooner we put him in the hospital, the sooner we can optimize his preoperative condition. You know how important that is. And you know the technology. Think about it. If your child had been born fifteen years ago, he wouldn't have a chance."

Stefan thought about this for a second. "How long will he have to be on antirejection drugs?" he asked.

"Probably all his life. It's a small price to pay."

"A small price to pay?" Roni blurted out, her face bright red. Until that moment she had been sitting in the corner of the exam room holding Nathan in her arms. "What about the psychological trauma he'll endure as you conduct your experiments? How much normalcy will my son experience in the first couple years of his life? What are the odds that he'll even make it off the operating table?"

The prevailing silence allowed normal hospital noise to filter into the room: clerks yelling for doctors, gurneys squeaking across the floor, and a tinny voice blaring over the intercom. The surgical resident shifted his body towards Roni. "Let's just get him there first," he said calmly. "We're talking about your son's life. We'll do the best we can. What else can you ask for?"

"Maybe just a little empathy," she said softly, and sat back down in her seat.

The surgery resident, young, tired, and probably childless, didn't respond. With a weary face, he shook his head and walked out of the room.

He had several more patient consults to finish, all at least as important as Nathan Spann's hypoplastic heart.

Jewish law and ethics, contained in the writings of the Torah and elaborated on in the Talmud, are quite clear on what binds a physician with a patient facing life-threatening illness. Life, a sacred gift to be preserved irrespective of circumstance, begins and ends under God's domain. No one—not doctors, nurses, or any other health-care professional—has the right to choose any form of euthanasia.

But the precise definition of human life is murkier. The Talmud states that abortion of a viable fetus is unlawful but not murder. The soul, or *nefesh* as it's referred to in Hebrew, doesn't enter the physical body until thirty days after birth, and therefore, even the killing of a newborn infant, though considered heinous, isn't a capital crime.

Was it this knowledge, or the fact that Jennifer was thirty weeks pregnant with our second child, that kept me from enthusiastically embracing the Spanns' argument? The way I saw it, Nathan, with no physical deformities or brain dysfunction, could undergo a heart transplant (though not a simple procedure by any means) that would ultimately save his life. If he survived the rigors of the transplant and then the prolonged period of hospitalization, aside from the lifetime of antirejection drugs he would be required to take, he would be, in all other respects, a normal child. He could be as normal as his brother Zachary.

Sitting across from the Spanns, I thought about this dilemma. I thought back to the first day we met and their lengthy interview of me. I remembered the personal background they had shared, their pointed and thoughtful questions, and the excitement that filled their eyes as they talked about being first-time parents. But those thoughts and that excitement was gone. Today their tone was somber and weighted with resignation, and their eyes, instead of appearing happy and hopeful, looked dull and weary.

"Have you completely ruled out the transplant?" I finally asked. "Is there anyone else, another surgeon, maybe some clergy perhaps, you'd like to talk to?"

"He has no chance at life, Ron," Stefan replied. "He'll be in the hospital for more than a year. He'll be invaded by tubes and wires. He'll be poked and prodded and injected full of drugs that have all sorts of evil side effects. Sometimes he'll be in tremendous pain and we'll have no way of knowing it. What kind of existence is that?"

"Remember what you told me you would do if Jennifer went into premature labor?" Roni interrupted, tears welling in her eyes. I remembered the conversation she was referring to—the conversation that residents finishing a rotation in the neonatal intensive care unit often had over drinks in some bar. The rare miracle notwithstanding, more often than not, saving infants on the border of viability with advanced neonatal technology left them with many untoward sequelae: blindness, brain damage, tracheostomy, stunted growth, and sometimes at the end of all the heroic measures—a not so pretty demise.

I remembered the discussion with my wife shortly after we found out we were pregnant: Why put an infant through unnecessary trauma and suffering when one could drive into the woods and let nature take its course?

Would any of us have really gone that far in those unlikely circumstances? Probably not, but I remembered the time I counseled the parents of a severely brain damaged seven-month infant to pull the plug on his ventilator. Born at twenty-six weeks and weighing in at just over two pounds, he had survived the throes of early prematurity only to be left with severe lung damage, blindness, and a brain that barely functioned. I remembered, at the time, taking the position on the side of quality of life, convincing the parents that letting their baby die was the best they could do for him.

"I know what you're talking about," I finally said. "But if the transplant is a success, Nathan will be normal. In three years you might have another Zachary."

The Spanns looked at each other for a moment before Roni turned to me with her response. "We talked about that last night," she said. "How much the two of them are alike. But then when we tried to convince ourselves to do the transplant we realized we were making a desperate decision. We're health-care professionals, we know too much. We know what it's like to let the technology monster destroy the human spirit. We know what it's like to make decisions based on data and statistics instead of feelings and emotions." She paused for a moment, studying my face, her eyes sad but resolute. "We're taking Nathan home with us to spend some time together as a family. If you aren't available to come to the house when he dies, we'll certainly understand."

The Spanns left my office an hour later. Roni sat in her chair nursing Nathan, while Stefan and I talked about resident and doctor issues: how to manage practice time and nights on call with small children at home. After they left I saw four children with uncomplicated ear infections, three with colds, and one older boy who was having behavioral problems at school. And before I left for the day, I turned my pager on indefinitely to fulfill the promise I had given the Spanns a couple of hours earlier.

Over the next few days several people contacted me. One of the cardiothoracic surgeons on staff asked me if I thought the Spanns were making a thoroughly informed decision, an anesthesiologist implied that Roni and Stefan were ex-hippies, and an ICU nurse told me they might change their minds if enough people pressured them. Every call boiled down to some variant of the same question:

What would it take to get the Spanns to reconsider?

I wondered if there was a reasonable answer to that question. Images of the Spanns floated in and out of my mind and I thought back to the day they first interviewed me and some of the questions they had asked. What is the current medical opinion on circumcision? Do you use a local anesthetic? Do you believe that infants feel pain in the same way we do? Do you counsel parents to use spanking as a form of discipline? Will you spank your own children? And the question that everyone asks: Why did you decide to become a pediatrician?

I became a pediatrician because I love to watch children grow, I told them. Seeing babies at two-month intervals is like watching them through a time-lapse lens, like being a parent without the responsibilities. And I chose pediatrics because it was a relatively happy field, mostly devoid of morbidity and mortality. One of the reasons I had not opted for a potentially more exciting and lucrative practice was because the average private practice child rarely develops life-threatening illness.

Although I did have my share of troubling moments dealing with death during my residency, private practice was mostly well checks, earaches, and behavior problems. Most of my time was spent plotting growth charts, pinning children down and looking in their ears, and trying to decide whether or not to use drugs for Attention Deficit and Hyperactivity Disorder. In four years I had hospitalized one child sick enough to be in the intensive care unit and had never had a patient die. I never had to inform parents that their child had an inoperable brain tumor or walk into a hospital chapel and watch two people my age grieve.

It was a Saturday morning almost two weeks after my consult with the Spanns that my pager beeped. I jumped from my couch as though I had received an electric shock and called the Spanns' house. "It's time," Stefan said, and after I told him I'd come right over, I rinsed myself off in the shower, brushed my teeth and had a quick cup of coffee. Not having done anything like I was about to do, I wasn't quite sure how long I would be gone.

When Stefan opened his door, he looked me up and down and without saying a word, stood to the side and pointed the way in. He was wearing soiled surgical scrubs that hung loosely on his thin frame and I noticed that his eyes were puffy and red, but dry. Inside, the apartment was divided into a kitchen, a dining room, and a small carpeted area where a well-worn couch stood in front of a thirteen-inch television.

The shades were drawn and a dim light from a small lamp in the far corner slowly brought the room's clutter into focus: Dirty dishes piled on the sink, clothes scattered on the floor, and a pillow and crumpled blanket lying on the couch. In the other corner of the room was an overflowing wood toy box painted with clowns and puppy dogs, with a Tonka truck and several Lincoln Logs on the floor next to it. A child's patent leather shoe.

As my eyes adjusted to the darkness, one of the bedroom doors opened and Roni walked out holding Nathan in her arms. It was obvious from her eyes that she, too, had been crying, but when she saw me standing there she gave me a smile as if I had been in the apartment for a long time. Then she nodded and headed for the couch, where she carefully laid her baby down on the middle cushion.

Nathan had been dead for a while—ashen skin, colorless lips, fingers curled and stiff—but when I kneeled at the side of the couch, I placed my stethoscope on his chest and listened. In the interminable silence, strange images flashed through my head. I saw a baby wrapped in newsprint lying inside of a trash bin, an infant that looked like a monkey hooked up to a respirator, and a fat Michelin baby playing in sand castles near a swing set. I saw a white, sterile nursery filled with plastic bassinets, each labeled in blue or pink, and each decorated with cardboard cutouts of stars and moons. I saw a lone crib in the corner marked DNP-DNS, the acronym for "Do not publish, do not show," a sign that the baby lying inside had recently been given up for adoption.

I stood up and wrapped the black tubing of the stethoscope around my neck, bundled Nathan in his blanket, and after gently picking him up, started for the door. "Thank you for coming," Roni said as I walked by. "Please make sure the pathologist who takes care of him handles him with kindness and compassion."

For the second time in two weeks, I was silent in response to her request, this time wondering if there was a medical school in the country that talked about kindness and compassion when performing a procedure as isolated and perfunctory as an autopsy. Certainly not in the days when I went to medical school.

I drove to the university hospital with the windows in my Jeep open, the air rushing in clean and fresh, uncharacteristic of Tucson's dry and dusty desert.

There was something different about its feel, not crisp and cold like the morning air in winter, nor thick and hot like the muggy blasts that begin in May and last through September. The air's texture resembled the mountains in the distance—sharp, clear and full of hope.

In the heavier traffic I looked at the people in the cars that passed and imagined what they thought as they glanced at Nathan, who was strapped into my daughter's car seat, eyes closed as though he were sleeping. Maybe they saw a father taking his son to the park for a walk, or to the mall to shop for clothes. Or maybe they noticed that my stroller was missing and that Nathan's color was just a bit too gray. What would they say if they knew the circumstances of Nathan's death and the car ride? Would my journey seem as strange and morbid to them as it did to me?

When I reached the hospital, I parked in the back and, after unhooking Nathan from his seat, stood next to the car holding him in my arms. I looked towards the hospital for an inconspicuous entrance. As a resident I had spent three years of my life walking in different doors at all sorts of odd hours to visit the pediatric wards, the intensive care units, and the newborn nursery. I remembered entering thousands of rooms, spending hundreds of nights on call, and answering innumerable middle of the night phone calls. And through all those memories I remembered one very special night: sleeping next to my newborn daughter in my wife's obstetrical room.

A friend of mine, a nurse who used to work in the neonatal intensive care unit, once explained that the reason she quit inpatient care was because she couldn't tolerate the grief—not just the sadness brought on by an untimely death, but the tragedy brought about by some of our medical achievements. "Technology has advanced faster than our wisdom," she had said, and as I stood holding Nathan, I thought about those tiny babies in intensive care that were barely hanging onto life because doctors had been taught to save life at all costs. Though I knew that hundreds of miracles were attributable to medical science, I also knew that some of those miracles came with a price, and I sometimes wondered if perhaps we shouldn't slow the machinery down a little and occasionally let nature take its Darwinian course.

I stood there staring at the tall cement building I knew so well. The Catalina Mountains rising up behind the hospital made it look tall and powerful, and as I watched an ambulance pull up to the back, my feet moved forward and I walked into the side entrance. From there I walked down to the morgue, which was in the basement, the third door on the right.

•

Ron Grant *left his pediatric practice in 1999 to write and earned an MFA in creative nonfiction writing from the University of Arizona. He currently teaches creative writing to medical students at the University of Arizona and is working on a memoir, entitled* The Other Side of the Curtain, *about his decision to leave medicine.*

The Last Train to Clarksville

A Journey through Breast Cancer Diagnosis

Cornelia Reynolds

❧

I sat shivering on the table wearing the regulation gown open to the front.

"Did you know 'The Last Train to Clarksville' was a protest song?" she asked. "The Monkees—you do know the Monkees?" I mentally pictured her as eleven years old when the Monkees were popular. "Well," she continued, "one of the places I worked at was Fort Campbell, Kentucky, near Clarksville, Tennessee."

My husband had inquired about her background. Our eyes met across the small examination room. Perhaps we were so aghast we looked interested. The surgeon who had taken only five minutes before predicting I would need a mastectomy was rambling on trying to make friends.

The Monkees, she went on to explain, were restrained by their management from doing anything political, but wanted to record an antiwar song. Their big hit, "The Last Train to Clarksville," was one of the few songs they recorded written by a member of the group. Its story of a couple parting at the train station is an invisible protest, because the young man's destination in Vietnam is concealed by the train ride to Clarksville, near Fort Campbell, the home of the 101st Airborne.

This anecdote was longer in the telling than the exam of my breast had been.

"Hello!" She exclaimed when she found the lump, palpating it briefly: "I can take this puppy out of there right now. Unless you're squeamish," she added in response to my look of alarm. "We could do it in the hospital on Wednesday. Then if it turns up malignant we'll do the mastectomy after the holiday."

Mastectomy? Did she think it was malignant?

"Well, you never know," she hedged, being politically correct, but yes, it seemed likely to be malignant.

Mastectomy? For a lump so small?

"Because it's positioned so close to the nipple," she said.

I left outraged by her hasty exam. But I was outraged with hope, fueled by the contrast between her predictions and what the radiologist had told me during an ultrasound examination the previous Friday: "This looks like a cyst, not a simple cyst, perhaps a hemorrhagic cyst, but it is unlikely to be cancerous."

Thus began my journey through the frightening landscape of breast cancer diagnosis. It's a journey still in the making.

Like "The Last Train to Clarksville," with its meaning hidden by the unnamed final destination, the unknown is central to this drama. My latest lab report concludes: "No malignancy was found. The results are not definitive."

Getting to this point has been an extended lesson in the business of cancer care—a part of the health-care establishment particularly besieged by the economics of managed care, the impact of an aging population, and the long-standing impasse in the war on cancer. I found that access to information affects access to care, and that economics and medical politics restrict patients' options. And, today, even with increased emphasis on patient participation in treatment decisions, doctors may still convey the attitude that all a patient needs to know is how to follow directions.

The patient's path demands a self-tutorial which includes, but is not limited to, the search for a doctor or team of doctors who will listen to and think in partnership with her. This demand is placed on a patient who may be in shock and is undoubtedly stressed by the need for immediate decisions about diagnosis and treatment.

In these circumstances the best help available was that of other patients, who told me their cautionary tales; recommended books to read; directed me to Internet sites; offered solace, and advice when asked; and generally urged me to question everything I was told and take charge of my own care.

I saw three surgeons before having my biopsy performed by a radiologist. Patients who had been rushed into fast decisions encouraged me to seek the ideal of having the same team from biopsy through treatment. Some saw three or more specialists before or after their biopsy, seeking a doctor and practice model with which they were comfortable.

I began to see this as an invisible protest march. In the doctors' offices, at the breast cancer centers, you see the parade of women — I was one of them — traveling with their films carried carefully under their arms, searching for hope and healing.

Among them I found a wealth of underground information to supplement, explain and contradict the medical establishment. These women created a culture of support and caring, a sustained and invisible protest to the rushed, insensitive atmosphere of much breast cancer care. In the midst of uncertainty, these patients provide each other the comfort of a listener's attention; the compassion of someone for whom the disease is an experience, not a concept; and the caring of another, a source of strength for whatever lies ahead.

My experience coincided with a string of conflicting reports on the value of mammograms in preventing breast cancer deaths. These began in late 2001, when Danish scientists dismissed five of seven landmark studies claiming that regular mammograms prevent breast cancer deaths. Confidence in mammogram screening has not recovered since, despite numerous expert panels which have each in turn announced that mammograms save lives and produced new and conflicting estimates of how many.

What I found in my diagnosis experience was that these circumstances of controversy, contradictory information, and conflicting recommendations extend deeply into the business of cancer. Doctors are well-intentioned but also hurried. They are untrained in patient psychology and driven by the conviction that early detection is the patient's best edge. The complexities of cancer combined with the subjectivity of doctor-patient relations fuel a brisk business in second opinions—and with it patients' autonomy and aggravations. One after another each doctor I saw contradicted the one before.

Too often patients encounter only conditioned responses from physicians. The surgeons I saw offered snap diagnoses, dismissed my observations of my own body, delivered recommendations as directives, failed to justify those recommendations, gave inaccurate or dismissive answers to questions—all the while pressing for instant decisions in response to their automatic diagnosis. This, based on a standard of care that says everything that is questionable must be biopsied immediately. Only physicians who saw their role as giving a second opinion had enough time, or used the word *recommend*.

This situation demands of patients an impossibly high learning curve for which little time is available. For many, the need for timely education must be filled by the community of fellow patients. Evidence indicates that breast cancer sufferers who receive group social support live longer. Perhaps this accounts for the spontaneous generosity that exists among women concerning breast cancer. In a short time I spoke with a dozen women, then several more; some called me—all of whom had experienced the procedures I was facing. Not all had cancer. One woman had biopsy surgery eight years in a row on successive anomalies found in her annual mammograms. It frightened her family so much that she stopped telling them about the procedures after the fourth benign outcome.

Patients' voices were more consistent, in marked contrast to the doctors. Their message: Be wary, take your time; biopsies are more painful and deforming than they tell you; decisions made now can ruin chances for later options; treatment can be as destructive as the disease itself; understand the downside as well as the benefits of every procedure; resist anyone pressuring you into having a procedure you don't want or don't understand; demand each action be justified and explained to your satisfaction. It proved a daunting assignment.

∽

When I first felt the lump in my breast, I considered myself an unlikely candidate for breast cancer. I am a fifty-five-year-old, postmenopausal woman of European extraction. Each of these factors pushes me up a notch on the risk scale. After gender (breast cancer occurs in men but accounts for less than 1 percent of male cancers), age is the predominant risk: 75 percent of breast cancers occur in women over fifty.

My focus, however, was firmly on the positive side of my risk profile. There has been no breast cancer in my family. I bore two children, the first before I was twenty; I nursed my babies; I had neither early onset of menstruation nor late menopause; I am not on hormone replacement therapy; I am slight of build (larger women are at greater risk); I have never smoked cigarettes; I drink alcohol moderately; I have eaten a low-fat, largely vegetarian diet for decades.

I considered myself well-educated on risk factors. I knew that nursing a baby before age twenty is thought to lower a woman's lifetime risk by 50 percent. I concluded I was well positioned regarding scientifically accepted risks, such as family history and lifetime exposure to estrogen. I thought my lifestyle lowered my risks further. I took my low risk profile for granted as protection when I irregularly examined my breasts in the shower, one arm, then the other, raised behind my head.

None of this came to mind, however, when I felt the lump in my right breast. Instead, instantly, a well of fear opened within me, my fingers jumped away from the lump. Fear brought my fingers slowly back, quickening rationalizations into place—or were they observations? I had felt a cyst before when nursing. This was not so different. It was close to my nipple, it moved freely, it was sore. *Why it's no lump at all, it's only a cyst. It will go away. I'm not a likely candidate for breast cancer.* I snapped my mind shut on it.

I had not yet learned that at least half of all new breast cancers are in women with no special risks.

I don't know how many days or weeks later my husband said to me in bed: "I've found a lump I don't like in your breast."

"Where?" I asked, putting my hand to his, letting his hand guide mine to show me exactly where, the well of fear striking open as if newly met. Later, answering my doctor's questions, I would remember the cyst I had so easily dismissed.

This lump was hard. I gasped, examining it. It was tender, but I know it's a misconception that breast cancers never hurt. It seemed free-moving, and apparently symmetrical, and small. Perhaps it's a cyst, I reassured myself. Whatever it is, it's small, I thought hopefully, unsure how small was small in a cancerous lump. The next morning I made an appointment to see my doctor.

I have a long-standing relationship with my primary care physician in rural northern California where we live. She supports and directs me in managing arthritis, diagnosed in adolescence, and fibromyalgia, a neurosomatic disorder with symptoms that include chronic muscle pain and fatigue. She knows these conditions influence other medical problems. She knows that I prefer the least invasive procedure, that I have a history of bad reactions to prescription drugs and avoid medications. She knows I am suspicious of mammograms for the radiation (cumulative exposure to radiation being an established cause of cancer) and, contrary to her recommendation, have mammograms with less than annual frequency. She knows I have felt railroaded by a cancer scare before, rushed by the threat of ovarian cancer into a full hysterectomy for a growth that proved benign. My recovery from surgery was protracted. Despite my qualms, she considers it her job to be cautious. "It could be something, it could be nothing," she said, and ordered mammogram and ultrasound examinations, arranging to have the radiology department of the nearest hospital fit me in that day, the Friday before Thanksgiving.

The hospital's questionnaire quickly focused my attention on risks: I've lived many years in northern California, a region with an above average breast cancer rate. I used birth control pills in my thirties; I used hormone replacement therapy (HRT) for over a year when I found my menopausal symptoms unresponsive to natural remedies and otherwise unbearable. The resulting summary on my mammogram chart read under Risks: "Postmenopausal, 1 year HRT."

A radiologist examined my breast with a small transducer, directing the ultrasound technologist to print several views. On the computer screen the lump appeared symmetrical, shaped like a bean, with a core at the nub. The radiologist said it was unlikely to be malignant. But if it were malignant, she reassured me, it was very small, only 5 x 7 mm. Lumps under 1 cm. are considered early stage, unlikely to metastasize.

She offered to perform a fine-needle aspiration to confirm that it was a cyst. Much of what followed might have been avoided had I already read the recommendation in *Dr. Susan Love's Breast Book:* "Any dominant lump should be aspirated before it's biopsied. It might be a cyst and surgery can be avoided." I had no map of this journey, but I already had an itinerary. My doctor had arranged a consultation with a surgeon for the following Monday.

A bilateral mammogram followed the ultrasound. A compression spot view taken of the lump area was particularly painful and left bruises on my breast. The radiologist reviewed the films to see that they were satisfactory. She told me the calcifications seemed unchanged from a mammogram two years before. Microcalcifications are tiny deposits of calcium that cluster around abnormal and dead cells, including dead cancer cells. Irregular, tight clusters in a single area may indicate cancer. A loose pattern, like mine, implies benign causes.

I was heartened by this information, but did not discount the possibility of breast cancer. Over the weekend I started reading Dr. Love's book, which patients recommended as a reference.

But I was unprepared on Monday. I was still in the chapter on diagnosis and the surgeon moved quickly to the topic of mastectomy. It was easy to resist her immediate excision biopsy. Her exam was cursory; she failed to read the radiology reports on either the mammogram or the ultrasound; she did not even look at the ultrasound films despite the fact the mammogram did not show the lump.

I asked why she didn't look at the ultrasound.

She said: "An ultrasound is useless unless it's dynamic."

I asked why she seemed so sure the lump was malignant, why it couldn't be a fibroadenoma, for instance, a type of benign lump I'd learned about over the weekend.

She said: "There are calcifications in the lump."

The mammogram report says of this: "Scattered punctate calcifications are unchanged [from previous mammogram] . . . [magnified] views of the region [of the lump] demonstrate a benign appearance. . . . The palpable nodule is not identified."

I asked if it might be a hemorrhagic cyst as the radiologist had suggested.

She said: "It's too hard to be a cyst. Besides, cysts are rare in post-menopausal women."

I asked her: "What if I don't do anything right now? What if I need time to decide what type of biopsy? How much time do you think would be reasonable?"

"That lump could metastasize at any moment," she replied quickly. "You will die if you do nothing."

So will we all, I thought in retort, but was stunned into silence. I knew I needed an education in breast cancer, and I needed another surgeon.

To her apparent credit, she offered: "If you don't like what I have to say, see another surgeon." She mentioned a breast specialist in a small city two hours away.

I told my doctor I found the surgeon hurried and cavalier, and we agreed I should proceed to the breast specialist.

My dissatisfaction with this surgeon went deeper than her devoting more time to chat than to her medical exam. What I found most unsettling was her lack of respect for my hesitation. I came to see the search for a doctor I trusted as a quest for one who offered me hope, for a benign outcome, for less than a mastectomy, for a healing recovery.

Like many other women, I lost a close friend to breast cancer, a woman in her prime, who never seemed to have an ill day—until she was treated for breast cancer. She died within a year, believing that she died from the chemotherapy.

I am struck by another irony of the Monkees' song—the refrain: "And I don't know if I'm ever coming home." Like the soldier going to Vietnam, the breast cancer patient doesn't know whether hers will be a death sentence, but the journey itself will be a life-changing experience.

The holiday intervened and the second surgeon would not see me for over a week. An eerie calm replaced the every-minute-counts pace. I used the time to talk to other patients, to continue reading. I was determined to have the least invasive procedure appropriate. I consulted a naturopathic physician and began a program of immune-supportive vitamins recommended for those at high risk for cancer. I hoped to strengthen my body for any surgery. I focused on visualizing a positive outcome. I also palpated my lump regularly and perceived it changing, sometimes softer and smaller, sometimes harder — changes characteristic of cysts. I began to accept my original feeling that my lump was a cyst.

The breast surgeon gave me forty-five minutes of her time, first carefully examining my breasts, my underarms and my neck. She read the radiology reports, looked at the mammogram, closely studied the ultrasound. She saw no other signs of cancer in her exam, she said. The lump itself was ambiguous. It was hard, but not as hard as most cancers. "Symmetry is rare in cancer," she added. "It might be a fibroadenoma."

She answered my questions at length but dismissed as subjective my report of changes in the lump. She advised an excision to remove the lump and a mastectomy if the lump was malignant.

Then I was dumbfounded to hear that she would not take me as a patient because she would not steal — she actually said *steal* — a patient from surgeon number one. I said I hadn't come for a second opinion, I had come for a specialist's expertise in recommending and performing surgery. She said I didn't need a specialist, surgeon number one was a fine surgeon. She was more than adamant; she gave me an additional ten minutes of her time to argue that she could not afford to offend the first surgeon, as they were part of the same regional medical community and regularly traded second opinions.

I couldn't win this argument; doctors have the legal right to turn down patients as they choose, except in an emergency. But she drew attention to my need for expertise. Unlike the previous surgeon, she discussed the significance of my general health and medical history for possible cancer treatment. She said large doses of cortisone administered for arthritis during my adolescence represent a cancer risk and predicted my history of drug reactions would make me a poor candidate for chemotherapy.

I asked her the question "What if I take more time before the procedure, how much time would be reasonable?" She replied: "I recommend a biopsy now, but it would not be unreasonable to wait a month in the absence of signs of growth. I would want to see that out of there by the beginning of the year."

With that she referred me on to yet another breast surgeon at a large medical institution, a great inconvenience due to distance. I wanted to jump off this referral train.

On the Internet, the War on Cancer is waged as a video game. Cancer Survival Rates unimproved since Nixon Declared War in 1971. Lifetime Cancer Risk approaching 50 percent (people are living longer). Evil Medical Establishment myopically fixated on Genetic Causes and Cure, with a not always benign Indifference to Prevention. In the midst of The Epidemic, in The Thicket of Claims and Counterclaims, patients circulate Healings, largely without the approval of the American Cancer Society or the Food and Drug Administration.

I preferred my pile of books, recommended by other women, some purchased at a community sale of used books. Here, the same information was available, in an environment as dominated by politics, contradictions and doctrinaire attitudes as the doctors themselves. I learned that among premenopausal women breast cancer is more rare, but likely to be aggressive when it occurs. Among postmenopausal women, breast cancer is more likely to occur but less likely to be aggressive when it does—something no doctor pointed out to me.

I discovered studies that challenged the effectiveness of chemotherapy and radiation in treating most cancers; I discovered the audacity with which the medical establishment waged war against pioneers of nontoxic cancer treatment and resisted innovators such as Dr. Judah Folkman, MD, whose discoveries led to the class of antiangiogenesis drugs (designed to starve a tumor of its supply of new blood vessels) now in clinical trials. These are not accounts to inspire confidence.

I handled with deference one among the used books, *The Breast Cancer*

Survival Manual by Dr. John Link, MD. A score of rough-torn yellow paper strips still marked pages throughout the book, raising the question whether the person who had placed them there had indeed survived. I read the marked pages looking for her story.

Dr. Link promises to "empower you . . . with the most up-to-date information available," kept up to date at his Web site. He reassured me: "The first information that I give a patient is that there *is time* . . . ," that a greater chance for a cure may be had by taking time to confirm the diagnosis, find an expert team and develop a survival plan.

I turned to patients to find a new doctor. Two unrelated people named the same surgeon in another city. He was described as trustworthy, gentle, and careful—important words in the patients' lexicon—and committed to minimally invasive procedures. He was, however, on vacation until after the holiday season. I made an appointment despite the wait.

A friend pointed out that I wouldn't avoid surgery by seeing a surgeon, and recommended another general practitioner—another long drive—for an opinion and referral. When I made the appointment, I was directed to bring all my nutritional supplements with me and to keep a food diary until my appointment.

This doctor spent an hour interviewing me about my medical history, reviewing my reports, and reading the labels on my supplements. He expressed surprise to find little fault with my nutrition. And he was hopeful I did not have cancer. But when I expressed reluctance to have the biopsy, he said: "It's too dangerous not to."

He recommended the same surgeon I was planning to see, but advised me also to visit a major breast cancer center that he considered committed to minimally invasive procedures with a strong research program on alternative cancer therapy. "They may not think a surgical biopsy is the way to go," he said.

In the end, my health insurance would not allow me to see both. I chose the large cancer center for its total program, despite the considerable distance to a major city. At this teaching institution appointments were booked a month out. The surgeon I eventually saw had the title Associate Clinical

Professor of Surgery. I had to interrupt her, as she came through the door already talking, to ask if I could record what she said.

She had reviewed a new ultrasound: "What you have is a cyst with a fibrous core. It's probably not cancerous," she said. "We are going to biopsy it to confirm that. This entails a radiologist anaesthetizing the breast and using a needle to get a few cells directly from the cyst."

From my research I recognized this description of a fine-needle biopsy. I was relieved to have come full circle back to the least invasive option. I thought I understood the procedure and asked only about a charge I'd read that the procedure could spread cancer. She dismissed this as unfounded. I asked whether cysts were rare among postmenopausal women. She said she had seen cysts in eighty-year-old women.

I asked: "What if it *is* malignant?"

"Details of any surgery would be determined by the results of the biopsy," she said. "However, this will not require a mastectomy."

This woman conveyed an authoritative manner, not without the appearance of bravado, and the impression that her time was limited. Her apparent expertise did not blunt my sense that I had not fully engaged her attention. But she said what I wanted to hear, and I needed resolution.

I put my mind to other things in the week before the biopsy. I discussed details of a fine-needle biopsy with my primary care physician, who had had the procedure.

Arriving at the hospital already tired from the long trip, I was shocked by the legal permission form that had "incision" in its title. I asked to see the doctor. What incision are we talking about here? The radiologist informed me a core biopsy was planned, one done with a needle so large that a small incision is required to introduce it into the breast. Unprepared for this, I questioned its necessity. The fine-needle biopsy takes a few cells out of the lump, this large-needle biopsy takes a small piece of tissue, in my case from the very small, suspicious core of the cyst.

I expressed concern about discomfort during and after the procedure. As a fibromyalgia patient I have found that medical procedures consume a great amount of energy and I recover more slowly than other patients. Focusing on the fine-needle biopsy, I had not read Dr. Love's description of the core biopsy as inappropriate for patients with arthritis in the neck or back, or anyone who may suffer from absolute immobility for forty-five minutes.

As it is, the radiologist convinced me that this was the least invasive procedure that would establish whether I had cancer. I was warned it might take two, even three tries to get enough tissue; that there could be bleeding during the procedure, bruising afterwards; and a lump that might take months to heal.

My breast tissue is dense, a disadvantage in this procedure. In fact, it took five tries, and over an hour and a half. There was considerable bleeding. The bruise lasted for weeks, as did the pain in my neck and shoulders. The lump has not healed yet.

Of course, the story isn't over without the pathology report. But like the traveler's destination in "The Last Train to Clarksville," the end of my story is hidden in obfuscation. The results were not definitive, but the recommendation was: "Follow-up ultrasound needed." The system has me and will not let me go. As scholar Ivan Illich describes the health-care business model: "The prior consumption of costly prevention and treatment establishes a claim for even more extraordinary care."

My journey may have crisscrossed northern California, but my passage was not unique. My daughter told me she thought I was exaggerating the brevity of my encounter with surgeon number one until, while doing research for me, she called an in-law who is recovering from breast cancer and heard the same story about her first visit with a surgeon in a distant city.

Health care in the United States is at a juncture marked by growing discontent among patients with the existing disease treatment model that particularly dominates cancer care. This model teaches us to distrust our observations about our own bodies, to underrate our intuitive feelings and healing capacities, and to surrender authority to professionals.

A new medical model may be emerging that acknowledges the personal aspects of health and healing. This model incorporates the evidence of anthropology that hope is an important treatment tool. It accepts the growing body of evidence for the mind-body health connection: that feelings and emotions influence health, and that support groups, like the much-studied Shanghai Cancer Recovery Club, can improve health. A recent series of advertisements in the Sunday *New York Times* for Memorial Sloan Kettering Cancer Center emphasizes nutritional and exercise programs, meditation and visualization, demonstrating that self-healing techniques are now entering the mainstream.

In this emerging environment, the doctor-patient relationship assumes increased importance. A review of curricula at the nation's medical schools reveals that physicians lack appropriate training in patient psychology. Indeed, the cancer surgeons I encountered demonstrated neither inclination toward nor experience in compassionate dialogue with patients.

Presenting an award, sponsored by the Fetzer Institute, to foster relation-ship-centered medical care, Dr. David Leach, MD, Executive Director of the Accreditation Council for Graduate Medical Education, emphasized that education and medicine have in common that "all cooperative arts depend on relationship." According to Dr. Leach, "The number one problem in medicine today is finding a way to create the space where relationships can happen."

In fact, the space where relationships can happen is well defined; it is the very space where relationships *must* happen, at the front lines, in the treatment rooms and offices where patients and doctors interact. Relationship in medicine doesn't mean making friends, though friendship may result; relationship means communicating and achieving understanding. In the cooperative aspects of healing, my experience is that the patients are leading the way.

•

Cornelia Reynolds writes and gardens in Elk, California.

Postpartum

Nancy Linnon

∽

ndrea Yates and I were pregnant at the same time. We had babies within two weeks of one another. We are both in our mid-thirties, white, of above-average intelligence. We both have husbands who love us and extended family members who support us. And last June, Andrea Yates drowned her five children in the bathtub, and I imagined crushing my beautiful baby's skull with a large, heavy book.

Andrea sits in jail, her children gone. I write this, my son happy in the next room, and so it appears we are very different. But as I pore over the stories in *The Houston Chronicle* about this mother, about her history before she killed her children, I know that our similarities could have continued. I know, because while others turn away from her story in horror or disgust, I turn toward it with an understanding so deep it frightens me. Like the undercover cop who gets too close to the criminal, I find myself slipping inside her experience, and it feels dangerous.

I sit at my computer searching online for more news reports, reading transcripts from the children's funeral, visiting the Yates family's Web page of pictures, and begin to feel eerily lost in my own home. I wander into the kitchen where my husband, Jesse, is cooking dinner while my mother-in-law takes lettuce and vegetables from the refrigerator and makes funny faces at my son, Jacob, playing on the floor.

"I was just reading the stuff about Andrea Yates," I say, leaning my elbows on the counter, resting my chin in my hands.

"Who's she?" Jesse asks absently as he stirs the pot on the stove.

"She's the woman who drowned her children . . ."

"Oh, please, I don't even want to hear about it," he interrupts.

My mother-in-law, who has abandoned the salad to join Jacob on the floor, tenderly brushes his hair from his forehead and says, "It's just unfathomable to me. I can't bear to hear about it."

I remain leaning on the counter, feeling a rush of shame for the morbid hours I've just spent obsessed with Andrea's story. And when I stand up and carry the lettuce to the sink, I also feel confused. These are the two people who saw me through the darkest days of postpartum depression, who watched my admission to the psychiatric hospital when Jacob was only seven and a half months old. Don't they realize how close I came, how serious it all was? Then, I immediately wonder if perhaps it *hadn't* been that serious. Denial can be comforting, and I silently wash and tear the lettuce and wonder if denial is what Russell Yates used to get through the exhausting days of raising young children. Did Andrea's doctors use it, too—the doctor who saw her two days before she killed her children, the doctor who reportedly leaned toward her and told her to "think positive thoughts"? Were the insurance companies, who cut short one of her hospital stays, in denial, or worried about the bottom line? I don't know. But I want to cry and scream as I make a simple salad—because no one understands how the trauma of the past months still threatens me. Because no one saved Andrea Yates, and no one saved her children.

I might have been Andrea Yates. I could say our paths veered sharply because my husband was more supportive, because I had one child and she had five, because I was already in psychotherapy when I had my baby, because I was not as sick as she was, because grace does not discern, because I was lucky. But that brings no comfort. In my mind, too much joins us. We were both convinced we were harming our children just by being ourselves. We both struggled to have people understand what we ourselves did not. We both tried to be stronger than we were able to be. We were both victims of disturbed hormones and faulty brain chemistry, of a managed health care system that believes psychiatric problems can be medicated away, and of a cultural mythology about motherhood that made our pain even harder to bear.

My therapist tells me that I was sick earlier than I knew and more sick than I realized. I walk home from the appointment and dig out my journals, dated December 2000 to October 2001. I shuffle through the pages to see if it's there: evidence that I was not in my "right mind." But mental illness is tricky. Even when you're medicated to "normal," the sick person you were is still inside you. And I'm there in those pages, hating motherhood, hating myself for hating motherhood, convinced that my son does not know who I am, feeling inferior to my husband in my ability as a parent, feeling guilty about the role my mother-in-law has to play, because I am not capable of raising my son myself. I am there naked and trembling and dying.

During my nine months of pregnancy, I doubt I was much different than most new mothers-to-be: I massaged my belly, I prepared the nest, I imagined intimate moments with my not-yet-born: breast-feeding by moonlight, tired but supported by a connection that transcended exhaustion.

I worked with midwives throughout my pregnancy and delivery—we met in softly lit rooms for appointments that were never rushed and that usually focused on the naturalness of childbearing. I told them my psychiatric history: two suicide attempts, on antidepressants for thirteen years, a grandfather who committed suicide, addiction throughout my family. I was off antidepressants during the pregnancy, but the midwives saw me stable and glowing, the wash of hormones keeping me afloat so well that I—and perhaps they—believed I would never have to resort to pharmaceuticals again. I wanted to breast-feed, and they encouraged me. I admitted my fears about getting depressed and they assured me there were antidepressants I could take while breast-feeding. I like to think that if I had known that my chances of falling into a serious postpartum depression were so high, I would never have breast-fed my son. But maybe I would have. Isn't breast-feeding what a loving, responsible mother does in the twenty-first century? Studies show the

benefits. I delivered my baby in a birthing center, fully conscious and unmed-
icated; I was determined to continue with the "natural" mothering process.

I call the midwife two weeks after having Jacob because I cry a lot, because
I feel overwhelmed, because I'm scared. All natural reactions to having a new
baby in the house, she says, friends say, strangers say. "Keep an eye on it," the
midwife warns, but keeping an eye on yourself getting depressed is like trying
to watch your hair grow—you know it's happening, but it's impossible to see
on a daily basis.

Soon after, when Jacob is three weeks old, I make an appointment with
the psychiatric nurse-practitioner who treated my depression for several
years before my pregnancy. When I enter the familiar waiting room—
husband, baby in baby-carrier, diaper bag in tow—I feel self-conscious and
afraid. I have spent years visiting this office, almost always sad, sometimes
despondent, always in need of support, and now here I am with a defenseless
baby. *What ever made me think I had the emotional capacity to have a child?* We sit
down, Jacob begins to fuss, I snap at my husband to do something. I haven't
breast-fed in a public place yet. I don't have my nursing pillow. How will I
get comfortable? What might be predictable fears for a new mom terrify me
into an edgy sweat. Eventually, Jacob latches successfully to my nipple, I
drape the towel properly so it covers my breast but doesn't suffocate him, and
I notice the receptionists smiling at me, approvingly I think. I feel capable
again, reassured. By the time I see the nurse-practitioner, my baby sleeps
peacefully against my chest.

"You certainly look bonded," she says, after I admit my fear that I'm not
feeling what I should be feeling as a new mother. "It's still early. Sometimes it
can take eight weeks to truly fall in love with your child, to be 'attached.'"

It is what I want to hear, and it's unthinkable that I continue to empha-
size how removed I feel from this adorable baby. As long as she uses the
magic words "attached" and "bonded" in regards to me, I figure I am imagining my own feelings. I leave with a supply of the antidepressant Paxil, just in

case, an antidepressant approved for breast-feeding moms that has never worked for me in the past.

I try to see myself as these medical professionals saw me: articulate about my symptoms, self-aware with a good support system. In short, a privileged but struggling new mother. I don't know if it ever occurred to any of them that I could hurt my child. They asked me about suicidal thoughts, but they rarely raised the specter of infanticide. My husband, my mother-in-law and my closest friends were all concerned about my safety, but I don't think they ever worried about Jacob's. Even if they had asked—are you worried you'll harm Jacob?—the truth would have caught in my throat, where it belonged. It is one thing to express self-loathing by wanting to hurt yourself, it is quite another to reveal that in a severely depressed mind, it is a short distance from suicide to believing your baby would be better off dead, too. Some must have known that postpartum depression carries with it the danger of infanticide, but perhaps there is a limit to what people can see, no matter how clear. Like the art that holds two pictures—one revealed by looking at the positive space, the other by looking at the negative. But you can only see one picture; the other has to be pointed out to you.

I put my brown bag of Paxil in a drawer, hopeful that the nurse-practitioner's prediction is correct: I'll feel like a better mother at the eight-week mark. And every time I successfully teach a class or spend an enjoyable hour with Jacob, I am convinced that the dark thoughts during my nights of insomnia are an anomaly. Often, like Andrea Yates, I think obsessively of knives: how big a knife I would need to kill myself, where on my body I would have to plunge it in order to die, whether I have the strength to do it.

One night, abandoning the bedroom where my husband and child sleep, I pace the house with my hands over my ears trying to silence the persistent desire to get rid of myself. I phone my therapist's answering machine at one

POSTPARTUM

A.M., thinking she'll be awake and call me back; I mentally run through a list of friends but reject calling each one, believing they wouldn't want to be awakened by someone being so overly dramatic. Finally, I wake my husband. He sits up with me all night, distracting me with talk about television shows and films we'd seen, in order to stop the images, in order to keep me alive.

During the day, I try to return to normalcy, even though it gets harder and harder. In the car, I find I don't know when to pull into traffic. I stare at the oncoming cars unable to push the accelerator; my perception is distorted, my reflexes are slowed. The Paxil, which I've begun taking, isn't helping, but I don't want to stop breast-feeding so that I can try other medications. It is not that I've experienced those intimate moonlit feedings I once imagined; I simply am convinced that my son will no longer know me if I'm not feeding him from my breast. Sometimes, when he is napping in his bed or already asleep in the early evening, I sit cross-legged on our bed, next to his, and fall into a kind of trance. I feel him float from his bed toward where the window meets the ceiling and then he fades into unfamiliarity, into nonexistence. Eventually, the phone rings or I hear a dog bark or someone talking in the other room, and I emerge again. I do not think of hurting him in these moments, but the lack of connection to him I feel, the fact that his drifting away actually feels comforting, fills me with unbearable guilt.

I stop breast-feeding at the four-and-a-half-month mark. The new medications — Lamictal, a mood stabilizer that I've never been on before, and Wellbutrin — appear to recharge my brain for a while, but it doesn't last. One Saturday morning, I attend a yoga class. I begin stretching, move into the postures, and desperation erupts. I start sobbing while doing the postures until finally I give up and lie flat on my mat. The instructor kneels down beside me, concerned. I whisper that I just need to rest, but in the stillness, images overcome me. In them, Jacob sleeps in the middle of our queen-sized bed and I reach to a shelf, take a hardcover book and smash it over his head.

I pick up my yoga mat, escape from the class, and drive home shaking. When I get there, I shut myself in my office and refuse to come out. Jesse is completely baffled by my hysteria, and I cannot explain. During all of these months, his love for me is one of the few comforts I have had. I am certain I will lose him if I expose the depth of my craziness. Maybe he could accept a lack of maternal feeling or thoughts of harming myself, but the images now forming in my head are evil, the antithesis of everything I'm supposed to be at this point in my life.

A good friend with grown children brings me a baby gift and a hot meal. She comments on how tired I look, but quickly turns her attention to the baby. She stays for an hour and when we're not quietly gazing at Jacob, we talk about mom stuff—pacifiers and feeding times and nighttime baths—and she remembers sweet stories from her early motherhood. When she gets ready to leave, she pauses just on the other side of the front door.

"Enjoy every minute, they grow so fast," she says.

I want to drop the last hour's façade and scream, "I'm not enjoying *any* minute," but that is not a mother's script. I know this, though I have never been a mother before. I absorbed it as a girl and then a woman, from playing house as a child and fighting over who got to be the "mommy" to being a thirty-something adult asked repeatedly and presumptively, "So, when are you going to have a baby?"

As she continues down the front porch steps, she stops to look back at Jacob and me through the screen door.

"You take care of yourself," she says. "These early months can be tough, but you'll get through it. It's all worth it."

I sit back down in the rocker, and Jacob begins to cry; I stand up, bounce him gently in my arms and feel doused in panic. I do not want to be with this child. I turn on a favorite CD and decide to sit on the porch in the early spring sun. The warmth feels safe, and I think I will be okay again, until I imagine myself throwing Jacob over the porch into the thorny bushes below.

It's curious to me how a culture soaked in talk of dysfunctional families, emotionally unavailable parents, and bad mothering makes little room for new mothers who find they cannot mother. It appears we can handle talk of troubled mothering in retrospect, but not in the moment. Few have the stomach to hear a new mother say, "I don't want to be with my baby." None of my friends coming to meet Jacob expected to hear that I was full of grief, that I wanted desperately to die, that I'd gladly give this child away.

Perhaps we can't bear to see unhappy new mothers because we can't imagine their babies' futures. Experts warn of the dire consequences for children of depressed mothers, but they rarely mention the mitigating effects an involved father or extended-family member can have. A child's future, it is suggested, depends on the "goodness" or "badness" of a mother.

Why couldn't I admit my anguish? Perhaps it was fear. Or shame. Perhaps it was as simple as not being able to admit the incredible failure I felt inside.

My therapist prepares to leave for a two-week vacation. I have seen her every week—sometimes twice a week—since Jacob was born, and in the worst times, I've kept in touch with her daily by email or phone. With her gone and the medication still not working, I can't stay safely at home anymore. The relentlessness of the illness exhausts me. And I am worn down by the pervasive guilt that I am not experiencing what I believe every mother before me has experienced. I am finally hospitalized at the end of July, after struggling with the depression for almost eight months.

I call my friend Kathy to take me to the crisis center late on a Friday afternoon. After the drama of the previous months, it is a decidedly anticlimactic moment that puts me over the edge: Jacob screams and flails when I'm changing him. I collapse on the floor with Jacob in my arms because I believe it is my fault that he hates to have his diaper changed. Jesse is at work, and my mind and spirit are so rattled that I know I can no longer care for this baby.

At the crisis center, I walk up to the front desk and stand speechless. I suddenly don't seem to know why I'm there, why Jacob has been left at home with my mother-in-law.

I stammer, "I'm depressed. I mean, I have a baby and I've been depressed since he was born." I hesitate. I'm not sure that is reason enough to be at a crisis center. "I'm suicidal."

"Have a seat," the man behind the glass tells me. "Someone will be right with you."

Kathy and I sit down and I begin to sob. Until this moment, I have been in perfect control. I even took a shower before I packed my things. But now it's as if all the months have collapsed on top of me and there is nothing more I can do but yell the truth from underneath them. I tell the social worker that I have thought of harming Jacob in the past. She asks for specifics and I choke them out.

"I don't have thoughts of hurting him now, though," I say, perhaps hoping for redemption. "But I want to die myself."

Later, she assures me there is no question that I need to be hospitalized. I feel relieved but am self-conscious about it: I shouldn't *want* to be hospital-ized, should I? I should have to be wheeled in, not pack and take a shower first. As sick as I've felt for all these months, I now wonder if I'm sick enough. The social worker tells me to go back to the waiting room while she calls around to see where there is an open bed in a psychiatric ward. She joins us a few minutes later with directions to a hospital on the other side of town and explains that I'll have to go through the emergency room in order to be admitted.

"Now, before you go to the emergency room," she tells Kathy, "the two of you should get some dinner. You will wait there a long time. A *long* time."

It's four in the afternoon. Then, she looks at me. "Do not leave, no matter how long they make you wait. Do not leave. You need to be hospitalized."

I think she must be exaggerating how long this is all going to take, but she is so emphatic that Kathy and I get a sandwich on our way. I nibble at mine in the waiting area of the emergency room and am acutely aware that I appear entirely normal. *Why am I here?*

When we're finally taken to a room, I believe the process will go quickly, but it has only begun. The nurse says I cannot eat the rest of my sandwich and takes my water bottle, too.

"We have no way of knowing if there is something harmful in this," she says, holding up the Bruegger's bag and the Arrowhead water.

She instructs Kathy not to leave the room unless she notifies a nurse first. The door must remain open and someone must be with me at all times. If I have to go to the bathroom, someone must follow me. The room is small, with no windows, but her words cause my claustrophobia. *I am not dangerous,* I think to myself. And the next thought: *If I'm not dangerous, I'm not sick enough to be here.* But they've taken my clothes and Kathy would never let me leave anyway. I stay and wait. Some of the time, Kathy and I try to watch the television hanging from the ceiling, but it feels silly. I need psychiatric medical care; television is too normal.

After a few hours, a black woman in jeans with bleached blond hair walks in, sits in a chair next to the bed, and begins firing questions: How long have you been depressed? Why are you at the hospital now? Are you actively suicidal? Do you realize you're self-pay and will be responsible for the bill?

At some point, I clear my head enough to stop answering and ask who she is.

"I'm a social worker and I'm here to see if you need to be hospitalized," she retorts. *Need to be hospitalized?* I feel as if I'm on the verge of failing a major exam. During my other depressions, I'd gone in the hospital unconscious — in retrospect, I believe, because it was so difficult to ask for what I needed without taking a handful of pills first. Now, the hours of waiting and the questions intensify my feelings that I am being dramatic. I am selfish. I'm not that sick, I just don't want to take responsibility for my baby. I am abandoning him.

When the social worker leaves, Kathy sees my distress, calls a nurse, and while they hold both of my hands, I cry and wait some more. In another hour or so, the social worker returns.

"Well, the doctor's signed off. You can go in the hospital." She sounds like I've been granted a luxurious cruise.

It's midnight by the time I finally enter the psychiatric unit, a brown brick low-rise built within the past year. The receptionist looks at my papers and asks, "Do you realize you're self-pay? It costs $850 a day to stay here." My eyes are red, my contacts so dry from crying that I can barely see. I tell her I'm applying for state aid.

"I have no choice but to be here," I add, doubting every word.

I'm not sure that any of the hospital staff knows I am a new mother. They do not ask about my baby. And when I mention to one of the social workers that I do have a baby, she begins to gush about her new grandchild. This is not exactly what I need to hear, but that is the tenor of the place. While they are aware I am being hospitalized for depression, no one ventures into what that might have to do with my being a mother. Everyone is very nice, but the biggest concern seems to be getting me insured so the bill will be paid.

During my third day in the hospital, my husband brings Jacob to see me for the first time, but they arrive at the same time the person from the state comes—unannounced—to have me fill out the medical assistance application. She has already, by telephone, asked my husband to gather bank statements, invoices, and receipts from my business and bring them to the hospital. This visit is to ask me questions about those documents. She stays for three hours, while I become overwhelmed by her questions. Later I will discover that you can make no more than four thousand dollars a year to qualify for that particular kind of state aid; it was evident from just one of my pay stubs that I would not qualify.

I wonder now about the nurses who ushered me into that meeting, who made eyes at my beautiful baby through the window but never suggested that the interview be shortened or rescheduled so that I could spend time with my husband and child. I was unable to act on my own behalf. They didn't do it for me.

I see three different doctors within the four days of my hospital stay. The first adds Effexor to my medication mix and decreases the amount of Lamictal I'm taking. On Monday morning, I meet with a female resident who increases the amount of Lamictal and adds a birth control pill. And the doctor who discharges me on Wednesday meets with me for no more than ten minutes, asks me without looking up if I feel well enough to be discharged, makes sure I will have all the medication I need when I leave the hospital, and quickly signs the papers.

Outside of these brief "medical" appointments, I drift through empty days punctuated only by meals and "medication distribution." On my first morning, an aide brings me a small cup of pills. I dump them in my palm and finger the unfamiliar white one.

"What is this?"

"Ativan. To help with anxiety. We give it to everyone."

"I don't really need it," I say, feeling a glimmer of my old self, wary of overmedication.

"Believe me, it helps your transition into the place."

The glimmer fades and I swallow the pill, hoping it will at least help me rest. But a psychiatric hospital is a terrible place to rest. I toss and turn for hours, my misery keeping my body on edge, exacerbated by my roommate's snores. Finally, I pull my blanket off my bed and shuffle into the hall. At two A.M., nurses gab at their station a few steps from my room as loudly as they would midday.

"I can't sleep because of the snoring," I say to the women behind the counter.

"I don't think there's anywhere else you can go," one nurse answers, looking at the other.

"She could go into solitary."

And I do, following the nurse through two locked doors and lying down on a metal slab with hand and foot restraints dangling from it. An impenetrable darkness startles me awake the rest of the night.

There is no professional to really talk to. One of the nurses tries to get me together with another patient, Carrie. She's a heroine addict in for court-mandated methadone treatment. She hopes to reclaim her two-year-old son from foster care.

"You might find you have a lot in common," the nurse says.

A social worker, with whom I meet privately twice, talks mostly about how to get me covered by insurance and gives me some handouts, after hearing my history, on being an adult child of an alcoholic. Later, she will draw a diagram of the public mental health system so I will understand how I will get my medication from now on.

None of these people are unkind. They make sure I am safe by marking down where I am every fifteen minutes. And I could go to them and insist they talk to me about my depression, about how I dread being with my baby, about how I believe I cannot live the life I now have. But I have trouble accepting all of that myself. How can I reveal these feelings to strangers when they don't ask to know? Worrying about the cost of the hospital is much easier than delving into the darkness of my psyche.

The day before I'm discharged, the resident doctor, who has shown genuine compassion for my illness, comes into my room to tell me that her residency at this hospital is over. I'm sitting cross-legged on the twin bed where I've been for more than an hour because I can't figure out what else I should be doing.

"You'll see another doctor tomorrow who will probably discuss discharging you, but I want you to stay as long as you feel you need to," she says.

I can barely hear her; she's talking so softly. I'm not sure why. My roommate isn't in the room, everyone on the ward is awake, and then it hits me: Doctors are supposed to discharge people, not invite them to stay. I feel dishonest, like I'm trying to get away with something. I hear one of the patients in the common room yelling at himself. Comparatively, I decide, I'm completely sane. I have a baby to care for. Enough messing around; I should go home.

I don't tell her any of this, of course, and as she prepares to leave, she says that she'll have my discharge papers ready for tomorrow's doctor should I want to go.

"You should stay if you need to, though," she repeats.

The next day, after seeing the discharge doctor, I ask for my red overnight bag out of lockup, where it's been held for safety reasons. I pack the few things I have in my room and walk out into the hallway. Several new patients have been admitted during the night, so it's noisier and busier than it's been the last four days. I sit down on the floor, my back against the wall, and watch. Nurses behind the main desk hand out Dixie cups of medication, patients wait to the side with questions: *When will I get to see my doctor? Can someone get my toothbrush out of lockup?* This is not a 1950s-era state hospital. This is not *One Flew over the Cuckoo's Nest.* But it is stark and impersonal and lonely. I sit on the cold tile floor of a long hallway with light green walls and not a single decoration. When Jesse gets there, he asks how I'm feeling, but I have no answer. I left my life for a few days, and now I'm going back. I'm not sure what, if anything, has changed. The social worker sees me as I'm leaving; I tell her my therapist will be back in town next week and she looks relieved.

A few weeks after my discharge, I believe the medication has begun to put a floor under me. But it's not just the medication. During the time I was in the hospital, Kathy, also a mother, visited me every day, listening to what I had told only my therapist: I hated being with my baby. She brought me oil pastels and we sat in the tiny, treeless walled-in courtyard and covered sheets of paper with color while I confessed every terror of the past seven and a half months. I wrote in a small "workbook," given to me the night I checked in, about how tortured I felt when I was with Jacob, how unhappy I was to be a mother. And although no one ever asked to read it, I offered it to at least one nurse, an important step in releasing my torment. I also admitted my thoughts and feelings to my husband, who, instead of recoiling, assured me that he loved me no matter what. Writing the unvarnished truth and receiving the support these two people offered, I believe, helped the medication start to truly do its job. Soon, my therapist would be back in town, and while I still had thoughts of killing myself, I had not had another image of hurting Jacob.

❧

The stories about Andrea Yates now chronicle her descent into madness. She was diagnosed as struggling with depression after the birth of her first child in 1994; she tried to kill herself twice—one time her husband found her scratching at her throat with a steak knife, another time she took an overdose of pills. She was afraid she would hurt someone, she told doctors, so she wanted to kill herself first. She reported hearing voices and having visions. She was described as "catatonic." She was hospitalized in 1999 and again in the spring of 2000. I read these stories and I wonder, *What more did this woman have to do?* If she had been an alcoholic or drug abuser, her insurance probably would have paid for twenty-eight days of inpatient rehabilitation. She could have gone to an AA meeting anywhere in her town. But a depressed mother was left with few options other than to take her medication and keep going as best she could.

I don't think Andrea Yates killed her children because she did not love them, because she did not want to be with them. Andrea Yates has a psychiatric illness, and she lives in a culture that does not support psychotherapy and that idealizes mothering to the point that reality is denied.

Even after looking right at it, my husband and mother-in-law could not allow their image of Mother to contain its opposite. Few people can. We would rather consider illnesses as horrific as postpartum depression and postpartum psychosis as aberrations. Andrea Yates is not the first woman to kill her children. Eight of the fifty-one women on death rows across the United States killed their children—and the majority of women convicted of infanticide are not sentenced to death. Approximately 182 children a year are killed by their mothers.

On this side of the most harrowing period in my life, I am angry. I am angry at the people who cared more about getting me insurance than giving me the help and solace required to heal a severe depression. I am angry at a health-care system that was eager to give me medication, but that seemed completely disinterested in the psychological and social aspects of my distress. I am angry at myself—for being complicit in a culture that discounted my history of depression in the belief that motherhood could cure all ills, that encouraged me to "enjoy every minute" of mothering when I was miserable, that attributed the symptoms of my serious illness to just "being a new mom," that sent me the message that my child was doomed if I wasn't a good mother. And alongside that anger, I wonder at my survival.

My now year-old son loves the water, and giving him his before-bed bath is one of my favorite times with him. With his wet hair reaching sweetly down his back, his eyes look even bigger. Naked, he seems even more whole and real and precious to me. I believe, despite what studies show about children of depressed mothers, that his life was barely interrupted due to the abundant time and care that his father, grandmother, and our friends were able to give him.

But there is never an evening when I don't think of Andrea Yates as I watch him smile and splash. I ache for her, for her illness, for her children, and I feel my brush with her fate.

•

Nancy Linnon is a freelance writer, editor, and teacher in Tucson, Arizona, where she lives with her husband, Jesse Vladimirov, and their son, Jacob. She is currently working on her MFA in creative nonfiction at Antioch University in Los Angeles.

Lessons from the Unlikely

Erin Newport

∽

When I was young, my mother read "The Pied Piper of Hamelin" to me. There were rats, a fat mayor, a piper dressed like a jester with bells, and a flute of some sort. I know my mother made her way through this story several times. It is the ending that I remember clearly. The piper comes to the mayor for payment and, when he is refused, leads all the children out of the village and into a secret entrance in a mountain. All the children, save one. He has a crutch. He wants to accompany the children into the side of the mountain, but he is too slow. The last picture of the story was of a little boy who sat, leaned on a crutch, and cried. It was haunting. It was at this moment I felt the Pied Piper as evil as the mayor, as filthy as the rats. He allowed someone to be left behind. To be left behind must be horrible.

In England in the 1800s, at the Royal Earlswood Asylum for Idiots, Dr. J. Langdon Down began making observations of patients who appeared to have similar physical characteristics—who seemingly belonged to the same family. He observed these features as straight, thin hair, small nose, almond eyes. He noticed that roughly 10 percent of the patients at the asylum possessed these characteristics. He termed them *Mongolian idiots* because their physical characteristics seemed to show influence from Mongolia, a region of east central Asia. Down's observations earned him a diagnosis given his name: Down syndrome.

He wrote in his "Observation on an Ethnic Classification of Idiots" in 1866, "I have for some time had my attention directed to the possibility of making a classification of the feeble-minded, by arranging them around various ethnic standards." He also notes as comparison examples of the "Ethiopian variety . . . presenting the characteristic malar bones, the prominent eyes, the puffy lips, and retreating chin. . . . The wooly hair has also been present, although not always black, nor has the skin acquired pigmentary deposit. They have been specimens of white negroes, although of European descent." His article appeared in the *Journal of Mental Science* in 1867, and his views were elaborated at much greater length in 1887 in a book titled *Mental Affections of Children and Youth.*

As hard as this information is to read, it would be doing Down a disservice not to mention that he used these arguments to prove some sort of *continuous* race, evidence of our human connectedness, evidence of common origin that randomly reproduces certain characteristics across the world. He promoted the thought that all humans were created equal. In the 1800s Down presented the institutionalized as compassionately and humanely as perhaps anyone of his generation. He observed that those he studied, those later diagnosed with Down syndrome, were "cases which very much repay judicious treatment." He noted several common personality traits: pleasant disposition, sense of humor and the "considerable power of imitation, even bordering of mimicry." He noted the short life expectancy that was "far below the average, and the tendency . . . to the tuberculosis which I believe to be the hereditary origin of the degeneracy." He was wrong about the tuberculosis, and it would be nearly a hundred years before the true cause of this condition was known.

In June 1993 my husband and I have our first child. He is born in the dark of early morning after a long and difficult labor, which begins a little before midnight on June 21st and ends at 3:21 A.M. on the 23rd. The room hushes, not all at once, but slowly, when he enters the world. His mouth is suctioned, and he is handed to the nurses. The doctor turns back to me, smiles gently, looks at me for a long time and then not again. The nurses glance at one another and proceed. I think my baby lovely, but the silence in the room tells me something. I watch as the nurses open his hands and look at his palms. They search and find a single crease, the transverse palmer crease, in his right hand. They whisper. A pink-and-blue stocking cap is placed on his head. He is wrapped in a blanket and is received by Tim, my husband. Tim's dark hair is a mess, his eyes moist. He smiles. He cradles our baby boy, proceeds to quietly and gently celebrate. I feel the guilt of an unthankful recipient, someone who has perceived the flaw in a presumably flawless gift. I lean to him and say, "Tim, I think something is the matter." He replies, "Nothing is the matter. He is perfect." I search the room again. I notice they have left us. We are alone when we name him: Peter.

It is November of 2000 and cold. I attend the TARC annual meeting and award banquet. As president of the operating board, I address the membership, highlight the successes of the year 2000 for this organization serving people with developmental disabilities in Shawnee County, Kansas. TARC stands for Topeka's Association for Retarded Citizens. It employs almost two hundred people and serves more than seven hundred individuals with delays in mental and/or physical development.

Most people refer to it now as TARC, because the word *retarded* has become ugly. It has been thrown around too many schoolyards, directed toward too many in conversations where it is considered a humorous put-down or a put-someone-in-their-place phrase. I hate to hear it used in these ways, but I use it to describe my son. People know what it means, what I mean when I say it. My reasons are practical, not callous. At the same time, I understand strong feelings can accompany something as powerful as a word that has begun to take on different and more sensitive meanings. I was once told the word *handicap* derived from the practice of the poor and often disabled begging for alms with cap in hand. *Retard* came from the musical term *retardatio*, which means to gradually slacken the tempo. When the word *retarded* was introduced, it was considered a beautiful term bestowed by a cultured society referring to a mental lessening of gain or progress, delay, slowness.

My son, Peter, hasn't received early-intervention services at TARC since he was three. He is now seven, and our three-year-old is almost ready to pass him up in size. He is tiny, one of the reasons it has been easy to integrate him into a kindergarten classroom of five-year-olds. He is thin, except for his belly. It protrudes slightly, due to lack of muscle tone, his stomach muscles not being strong enough to hold everything in nice and tidy. As a result his torso is the shape of a kidney bean: a bit of an arch in the back, fullness in the front. His eyes are a mixture of blue, from me, surrounded by tinges of brown, from Tim, and have been framed by little golden rims since he was a toddler.

After Peter is born, he is relocated to the neonatal intensive care unit, where he receives medicine to rid his lungs of fluid. I spend my days at the hospital. The nurses encourage me to take a break, get some fresh air. I am not allowed to feed him yet; his stomach receives my milk through a tube inserted in his nose. Yes, they all agree that a walk will do me good. I exit the hospital to the rain and drizzle that has plagued our Kansas summer of 1993. I am drenched by the time I cross 10th Street to the Topeka and Shawnee County Public Library. I make my way to a computer that the librarian has told me is dedicated to accessing a medical database. I begin printing out everything I can on Down syndrome. As the pages pour from the printer, I begin to read. Most of the information is outdated, though I don't realize it at the time. One of the first facts I stumble upon is a 1975 poll revealing that 77 percent of American pediatric surgeons favored withholding food and medical treatment from infants with Down syndrome, leaving them to die rather than sending them home with parents or families. I leave the library and a busy printer still spitting out the dreadful stuff. I make my way back across 10th to the hospital — to the NICU. I enter soaked and winded, stutter when I tell them I have decided to come back early. I decide to stay with him at the hospital as much as possible.

In the days following Peter's birth, I remember that during our engagement Tim told me he had always thought he would one day have a child who would be "slow." He wanted me to know this, felt the disclaimer necessary. I think it is ironic but perhaps no more so than the fact that Down's grandson and namesake was born with Down syndrome. Records of the grandson, John, describe him as a lovable person and a good billiards player.

Approximately two weeks after Peter is born, I receive the confirmation that he has Down syndrome. I take the call from a phone in the NICU. I ask for a copy of his *karyotype,* the picture of his chromosomes that confirms the diagnosis, a word recently added to my vocabulary. It will be sent to me.

Tim and I met in college in the late 1980s. He looked fifteen at best. He has matured and now looks at least twenty. At first I wondered what to make of him. He was lanky and thin, possessing an unusual amount of energy and talking in a rapid, Southern dialect. Long before we began dating, he began walking with me at night, around the brick lanes that circled the campus. I stared in disbelief as he repeatedly fell into hedges or tripped over curbs, once rolling down a hill. Later he would tell me how nervous he was during the walks of those years. It should have been an indication to me of his attentiveness to a fault. From the very beginning, he was willing to forfeit some awareness of his own two feet and various pedestrian obstacles for my sake. But back then I just thought him clumsy and told him so on several occasions.

I have since pocketed dozens of these attentive examples in my memory: Tim rubbing baby lotion between each of Peter's toes, his waking each night to change baby diapers, and still waking again when one of the other kids has a bad dream or needs a drink of water. There are the nightly foot rubs and the surprise trip to Chicago to attend a Norman Rockwell exhibit. He trims my father's trees and hedges, runs to the store for my mother, is even attentive to the neighborhood kids. More than once I have opened my front door to a group of kids asking me, "Can Tim come out and play soccer?"

I sit in the lobby outside the neonatal intensive care unit, a blue room with faux antique chairs with high backs and carved wooden legs. The furniture seems out of place next to the stainless steel sink that runs the entire length of the wall to my left. Instructions on how to sterilize your hands to the elbows and directions to the sterile gowns are provided above the sinks. All visitors must wash before entering the unit, which is just past the electronic glass doors.

People want to know what caused it and whether or not it runs in the family. My aunt visits me at the hospital and tells me, "Well, you know, — — is pregnant now. I sure hope she doesn't have one." I tell her I think it is unlikely. I try to be reassuring.

Peter remained in the hospital for almost three weeks. I arrived home from days spent with him to find my house clean, dinner fixed and warm on the stove. Most of my family and friends proved invaluable. I found their questions and comments timid and sincere and careful. I was grateful, and they were lovely. I don't remember the specifics of the questions now, but I do know I replied by regurgitating all the facts I knew, the facts that connected me somehow to the baby in my arms. I told them that approximately 1 in every 800 babies is born with Down syndrome. I told them the chances of having a child with Down syndrome increases as maternal age increases. A woman age forty has about a 1-in-100 chance of having a child with Down syndrome. The chance of my having a child born with Down syndrome in my early twenties was about 1 in 1,450. I sketched out dozens of illustrations of chromosomes, feeling relieved and gratified as I drew them. With a pen or pencil or crayon on a piece of scrap paper or on the palm of my hand, I drew and drew, like a mad geneticist. I, who blush so easily, attempted to give all who desired it access to the explanations of the very personal, and now very public, conception scenario.

I have always been an art enthusiast. As I begin to educate myself on Down syndrome, I notice and store the bits of information regarding Down syndrome and its portrayal in art. What did societies formerly do with people like Peter, people who were different? What place did they find in culture? Their representation in art might tell me. I search for evidence of compassion or tolerance. Finding examples would be treasure to me. I want to know if we were capable of seeing past the surface. I search for the exceptional specimen in a painting, or even a photograph, so I can examine the artist's choices, explain and reveal his or her desires, name those things worthy and sought after. I take great delight that some of Velazquez's favorite subjects were the dwarfs in Philip IV's court, whom he portrayed as full of human dignity.

Several medieval and Renaissance artists are rumored to have used children with Down syndrome to portray the infant Jesus. I can find no definitive truth, no scholarly articles or art criticism that addresses this claim. I say there is no definitive proof *in writing,* but there are the paintings themselves, which one can view and then decide. Bellini, Brueghel, Reynolds have been cited in various Down syndrome publications as using models with Down syndrome, but it is the works of Andrea Mantegna that are particularly convincing. His Madonna-and-Infant paintings are so psychologically connected — a child wrapped in the arms, the body, of a mother who seems to protect it from all angles. It is a child who is vulnerable that Mantegna presents. It is not only this portrayed vulnerability that makes me wonder, but the characteristics, the features of the infants of Mantegna. It is the almond-shaped eyes, the open mouth, the tongue slightly protruding, the placement of fingers and toes that appear respected and reproduced from a child with Down syndrome.

I receive Peter's karyotype in the mail. I have waited a lifetime for it. I look at his chromosomes, lined up and numbered on paper, so tiny, so powerful. The three chromosomes labeled "21" are a quarter the size of chromosomes 1 through 12. I think them rather sumolike in their stance; the bottom half of the X looks like two thick, stubby legs, slightly spread. But the top half contains almost no genetic material at all, looks like a set of antennae topped with tiny, clenched fists. I read that these "fists" have a magnetic quality, which is possibly what causes the chromosomes to not separate correctly. I place the karyotype in Peter's baby book, next to the strangely familiar sonogram images: a tiny baby with clenched fists.

I become crazed with trying to understand and explain this genetic occurrence. My husband and I teach ourselves basic genetics, begin to understand how this small amount of extra genetic material on chromosome 21 affects each of Peter's genes. This chromosome starts a progression of developments that eventually can be recognized in the palm of his right hand, in his facial features—upward-slanting eyes, small ears, button nose, mouth seemingly too small for his tiny tongue, teeth—the shape of his head, his low muscle tone, and the compromised respiratory system that was rightly noted but wrongly diagnosed by Down in the 1800s as the source of the syndrome.

Tim and I take our baby home. He never cries, so we string bells across his bassinet so we'll hear him when he wakes and squirms. We train ourselves to hear little bells that jingle in whispers. We tune ourselves to them, hear them from anywhere in the house.

My job working with the long-term unemployed expires with its grant funding five days after Peter is born. After he is home, I make a trip to the unemployment office to apply. It is located on the floor above the one I occupied just a few weeks earlier; I shared a break room with the people who will be processing my papers. It is awkward. News has spread of Peter. They pass over my paperwork for close to an hour. It sits in the rack, and I watch as it is pulled out and my name on the application is read. My acquaintances nervously scan the chairs for sight of me and quickly put it back. I assume they are now appealing to the floor manager to process my papers. She rarely processes papers. She wears big, round glasses and stiffly says, "Well, you've certainly lost some weight since we saw you last." She turns red, wipes her palms on her dress. Peter is never mentioned, and I feel sick about it.

As I exit the building, I almost knock over a woman taking a smoke break. I recognize her face but don't know her name. She pulls the cigarette from her mouth and says, "Hey, we heard about your little guy, and we're rooting for you." I mumble some sort of thanks and hurry away as I begin to cry. What I really want to do is run and throw my arms around this lady. I want to reach out and grab her words, which have already scattered into the air. I want to press them in Peter's baby book, keep them forever. I remain deeply indebted to those brave enough to address my having a child born with a disability. Whether they did so tactfully is not my concern. It is their effort and courage I cherish.

After Peter is born, an acquaintance tells me, "You know, it is really too bad you and Tim can't have any more children." This is news to me. I wonder if my ovaries have betrayed my confidence, told her something that even I am not privy to. Then it dawns on me. After our having a child with a disability, it is assumed we are done. She might just as easily have said, "Folks, I think your turn is up." In a sense Tim and I together are considered a bit of a liability. Nonetheless we continued to have children, to the world's dismay and to the disapproval of a few.

Both of us wanted brothers and sisters for Peter, and it was interesting to come across the writings of Down that describe his own desires. The patient, he said, "should be rescued from his solitary life and have the companionship of his peers. He should be surrounded by influences of art and nature, calculated to make his life joyous, to arouse his observation and to quicken his power of thought."

Peter is the only boy in a house full of girls. "What we have to put up with . . ." my husband tells him. "We need to stick together," my husband tells him. But he is lost to us women, our influence too strong. He begs for fingernail polish when we pull it out to do our own nails; he is one of the loveliest in the long gowns worn during dress-up. (Gowns are more fun than trousers, so plain, so ordinary.) My husband is fit to be tied, tries to instill in him the right and privilege of being able to pee standing up; still Peter insists on sitting. I am thankful.

By the twelfth century, paintings were used as the foundation for interpretation of higher spiritual truths for the nonliterate, and perhaps these values were making themselves apparent in content as well as subjects. Mantegna is known for historical accuracy with a glimpse of bitter reflection. Yet he is known even more for extreme interpretations shedding light on qualities that are in turn tragic and ironic. If Mantegna possessed a social awareness unequaled among Renaissance painters, a compliment he is given freely, it is not so difficult to believe that he would have chosen children with Down syndrome to portray religious figures in art. Children with Down syndrome are often identified, naively I think, as angels or as possessing standards of divine beings. I agree with neither. However, people are driven to locate us in crowds, to make their way, out of their way, to tell us about how they are related to someone with Down syndrome, to tell us stories of their experiences with people with Down syndrome. They relay how they identify something special and unique—we have identified it ourselves. It is obvious that these children would be ideal models, perhaps not physically, but spiritually, for Christ.

Tim and I have noticed that children with disabilities are not chosen to sell toys, are not in commercials, are not the subject of Anne Geddes portraits. They are scarcely represented in any visual art form now. It is only after Peter that I discover the specifics of the subject in Andrew Wyeth's painting *Christina's World*. It is often perceived as a romantic picture of a young woman lying in a field of scattered yellow flowers. It is actually Christina Olson, a neighbor of Wyeth's in Cushing, Maine. She is middle-aged, disabled by infantile paralysis, stranded by the family's burying ground. She is alone and unable to get back to her house, which is small and brown in the upper right-hand corner of the painting. It is a picture of abandonment and despair, but one would never know. So far are we removed. We see vulnerability so seldom we have difficulty recognizing it. It is frightening for me to think that one day we might lose our appreciation of the weak, lose the sense that our own strengths are to be used for others, assume that our abilities are only for our good and for our gain. It seems that the weakening of this part of our awareness will result in the recession of our collective compassion. I imagine it glistening on the corners of our thoughts, then proceeding on to the furthest spots of our memories. It will blink and teeter, will be extinguished and be lost forever.

In the early 1970s, photography had found subjects in people with disabilities. Photographic essays were largely extrapolated from institutions that had separated us, hid from us our children born with exceptions. In 1970–71 Diane Arbus published an untitled series of photographs in *Aperture.* They feature the tenants of a mental institution, many with Down syndrome. Many of the photographs appear to have been taken around Halloween. Women in fancy hats and bonnets carry handbags; thick stockings cling around their knees. They smile in front of brick walls that feel of institution. Another photograph appears to be of a sort of parade. A determined and grouchy woman in a nightdress faces forward and marches; her hand clasps a young man with Down syndrome. He has a painted, handlebar mustache and looks at the camera. A woman in a wheelchair holds a mask (of a witch, I think) over her own face.

I can't figure these pictures out. They are surreal and feel itchy on my eyes. Frankly they are frightening, and I wonder, What are those women in swimming suits doing out on the lawn of a mental institution? Isn't it October? Is this Halloween or is it something else? Something scarier? Do these pictures document a collection, an amassing of difference, of so much difference it created a different world? Such a different experience. It leaves me not knowing at all how people of this time regarded those with disabilities. I think I begin to see the separation—of not knowing where these people go. It feels like a circus.

A few years ago, I read that Arkansas State Health Director Joyce Elders, in testimony before Congress in 1990, expressed support for abortion of Down syndrome fetuses as public policy. "Abortion has had an important, and positive, public health effect. . . . The number of Down syndrome infants in Washington state in 1976 was 64 percent lower than it would have been without legal abortion." I read it again to be sure that I understood it right. The truth of the matter is so casual, so hidden in the middle of public policy that it is easy to breeze right over it, not realize just what Joyce Elders was proposing, supporting. It feels like a moment in the movie *Life Is Beautiful* where people at a dinner party are discussing mathematical story problems being taught in the schools. The dilemma presented to the children, relayed through their dismayed parents, is something like this: If 600 Jews are sent to Auschwitz and 325 Jews are sent to another concentration camp, how many Jews will be killed in the concentration camps? When the movie's heroine agrees that this is horrible, the others in the party say something like "Yes, how can my child be expected to do these advanced mathematical calculations? He is only in second grade." And there it is. The ugly truth about what Germans thought of Jews in the 1940s. And there it is. The ugly truth about what my culture thinks about people with Down syndrome in the 1990s.

People often ask me if we knew Peter would be born with Down syndrome. It is now possible to tell all sorts of things about unborn children. People can screen for gender and a variety of diseases. Tim and I checked for nothing but a heartbeat. It was enough for us. When we were pregnant with each of our other children, we were always offered the "opportunity" to find out more about them. We declined.

It seems a grand pursuit to explore our origins, to contemplate our beginnings, to speculate. We, evolved of goop and goo; we, formed from clay. This desire is one of many to examine ourselves closely, our makeup. It is in some sort of self-interest that we question where we came from and how we came from it. We seek what the world looks like up close, the visuals of our smallest components. It begins as a child with a fascination with the less-obvious parts—in between the toes, elbows, the inside of the nose. These odd and uncoordinated exercises of examination are the precursors of moving closer.

In sixth grade I study protozoa, small, single-celled, aquatic organisms, a phylum of the animal kingdom, reproduced by binary fission. Single-celled organisms we are not. We are a collection of sorts, of different sorts of cells, which differentiate somewhere in the evolutionary process of the womb, become white blood cells, red blood cells, bone cells, brain cells. Mr. Kralik introduces my sixth-grade class to the proper care and use of the microscope, shows us how to mount specimens on our slides carefully to avoid the air bubbles that would complicate our observations. After all is ready, a drop of pond water is placed on the slide. I move my eye to the lens of the microscope. I immediately zoom in for a closer look at a world newly discovered. I feel like Columbus. These protozoa are akin to the parts of me that I cannot see, do not see, all that is there in the layers underneath my skin.

I am reminded of Dr. Seuss's *Horton Hears a Who,* and I imagine one newfound protozoan a Who at heart. He is trying to communicate with me; he senses my observations, responds by squirming. He, she, it wants to say something but has no mouth that I can see, has nothing by the way of skin or features, though it does somewhat resemble an ear. This is one of the living, breathing organisms that end up everywhere, in everything, on the end of my fork. This close-up is intriguing. I want to push my way even closer, to squeeze in for a better view.

After Peter is home, I take long, close looks at this little baby, my specimen of study. I examine his eyes: their slight slant, the small folds of skin, called *epicanthal folds,* in the inner corners. His nose and its flat bridge are textbook. I read up on Peter's hand. I see for myself what the nurses were looking at. In my own cupped hand, two creases. One begins above my thumb and curves down; the other, just under my pinky, curves up across my palm to my middle finger. They arch slightly and miss each other. Peter's creases collide.

There are the Brushfield spots in his eyes, tiny, light dots surrounding the pupil in the blue and brown of his iris. It is as if a paintbrush has dabbed his eye and lifted out the color in little, bristle-fine spots. I take note of his small ears, which sit lower than normal. The space between his big toe and the four smaller toes is a bit wider than usual. I especially notice the muscle tone, which Down mistook for skin that did not retain its elastic quality. Peter is wobbly and weak. He does not hold up his own head until he is almost ten months old. He does not walk until he is two.

In 1959 Jerome Lejune, a French cytogeneticist, discovered the presence of an extra chromosome in individuals with the physical characteristics observed by Down. It wasn't until later years that scientists knew where the extra chromosome belonged, on the twenty-first pair. Our genes—the blueprints of life. From our rods of chromosomes we can trace our sex, eye color, skin, hair texture, voice. Our genes determine the way we begin and sometimes the way we die. The sperm offers a chromosome, and the egg offers one, as well. It is the moment of meiosis when the chromosomes split exactly in half, offer themselves, conceive something new, duplicate. The new cell divides into two; those divide into four, then eight, then sixteen, and continue to divide for nine months and then throughout our lives. We are millions of cells made from the original, regenerating and duplicating over and over. What we see around us are the results of twenty-three pairs of chromosomes, big and small, striped X's and Y's that contain the whole plan of the world.

It is at the moment of meiosis that the individual with Down syndrome inherits the extra chromosome, through a faulty chromosome distribution. The chromosomes don't split exactly in half; they fail to separate or disjoin, and the pair becomes lopsided and heavy with extra material. The pair on the twenty-first chromosome sticks together, and the extra chromosome becomes part of the new, living embryo. And as it grows, the extra chromosome is replicated and transferred to each new cell. Three chromosomes on the twenty-first pair equal *trisomy 21* for 95 percent of the babies born with Down syndrome. The two other types are *translocation,* when part of the twenty-first chromosome breaks off during cell division and attaches to another chromosome; and *mosaicism,* when the faulty cell division occurs after fertilization, resulting in only a portion of cells containing the extra chromosome.

Peter is a ghost every year for Halloween. We throw out all sorts of ideas every year: a pirate, a cowboy, a scarecrow. He will have nothing to do with our suggestions. He chooses the garb of a ghost this year again and becomes a different kid, with not-so-Casper-like qualities. Once the homemade sheet costume is slipped over his head, he becomes hunched. His hands are raised. His vocabulary is reduced to "Boo!" with varying inflections and accents. He considers his frightening new abilities, begins slowly sneaking up on people from ten to fifteen yards away. His approach takes a quarter of an hour. We have ample time to plan a surprised response.

I wonder, Where is the place for people like Peter in this culture? How will he be preserved and presented to those after us? I wonder if a child with Down syndrome could even be imagined in the arms of a Madonna now. Public records show that only one in ten couples will choose to have a child with Down syndrome if the amniocentesis tests positive. I wonder if people will know what a child with Down syndrome looks like fifty years from now, ten, five. I face my culture and my government, and it seems as if I am meeting an armed Diane Arbus in a dark alley. She wields a camera in one hand and a blunt object in the other.

When Peter was about three and Maggie a newly walking toddler, a woman singled me out at work. She was in her mid-fifties—a different generation, granted. She told me that she had heard I had a child with a disability and another, younger child. She told me she too had a son with a disability, long ago. She kept him for a while, but when she became pregnant with her second, he was just too much. She sent her one-and-a-half-year-old child to an institution. It was not the ending I expected, and I wondered why she was telling me this story. I thought about how she still carried him with her, not in the typical way a mother carries her child, but in memory, which is often much heavier. In telling her story, she revealed in a generous and selfless way so much of herself. I knew she was telling me that she was like me. She wanted me to know that she had experienced something of what I had experienced. I knew she was seeking a connection. I found it hard to appreciate.

I nodded and listened and thought, with a nasty bit of self-righteousness and fear, *No, I am not like you.* I thought her selfish and so preoccupied with the newness of another life that she forgot the value of the child who called her mother first. Never did we consider not taking Peter home. Never did we think that those who came after him would be more valued. Never did we think we had to choose among them, like worn-out blankets or winter coats, which was worth keeping and which was not. I wondered if her second child and her third and those who followed ever went to sleep wondering if tomorrow would find them replaced by someone or something else.

Perhaps I react too strongly. Still, I wish people sought out the part of themselves that overcomes, that embraces the struggle as a means to learn about life, our responsibility in it, to it. I claim this as my passion. I say it is right and grounded. I say with fervor that one should react strongly to all that grates against the conscience, and I say this because my stakes seem higher. There are those who will argue that our sense of right and wrong is a given part of us, something we share, like arms and legs. I suggest it is a muscle and must be exercised. The voice of conscience, unused and unpracticed, easily becomes inaudible, like the quiet tinkle of little bells strung across a bassinet.

I feel a great deal of gratitude to TARC, which was established in 1954 when parents found themselves and their disabled children shut out of school systems, day-care centers, society and privilege. They began raising money by hosting bake sales, making private donations, selling Stanley Wax, and at the end of their first year, they had eight hundred dollars to serve their children.

Tonight the membership listens as I tell them that inventing a future is a lifetime of work. I look out over the dimly lit room at the numerous round tables, which hold cacti of various sorts meant to add a Southwestern quality to the Western theme of this year's meeting. Staff bustle about with blue bandannas tied around their necks, pouring tea and delivering the dinner salads. I look into the faces of the members and see their age. They've heard what I have to say a hundred times before but listen kindly. As I address them, I am thinking about how I want to persuade them that the young parents of today will not drop the ball. But where are the young parents?

I think about how Tim and I fought long and hard to get Peter into our neighborhood school. The meetings were brutal, especially for Tim and me, who consider ourselves "nice" people, "reasonable" people.

We arrived at the first official meeting to be told that Peter's teachers were recommending he be placed in a classroom where only children with disabilities would attend. We expressed our strong feeling that Peter should attend the school his sisters would attend. We explained the value of his attending school with "normal" kids, thinking this arrangement would be good for his language and for his social skills, not to mention the academics. We were told we were "valuable members of the team," but it was the recommendation of the team that Peter be moved to the secluded classroom. We were told we could appeal the recommendation but that the administration would not side with us. Tim got up, told them the meeting was over, thanked them for their time.

Immediately Tim and I shifted to business mode, something we have learned we must do to remain effective advocates for our child. To the meetings that followed, we brought copies of the IDEA law and encouraged the staff and administration to reconsider their recommendation. We pointed to the parts of the law where their actions could be considered illegal. "No hard feelings," we told them. "This is just business." But it was actually much more than that, and we all knew it. Several parents opted to accept the recommendations presented by staff and administration instead of going through the whole process of appeals. But in not advocating, it seems they are laying waste to all the hard work and gains that are laid at their feet. Peter is allowed in the schools; there was a time when parents couldn't even expect that. I worry that many young parents have not been educated about the efforts of these people I address, don't realize they must get involved and advocate, don't realize they ride the backs of those in this room.

Peter insists on making his own breakfast. When he was six, I thought it would be a good thing for him to learn, so I bought some toaster waffles. We learned how to operate the toaster, where to find the butter, syrup, utensils. It has been a thorn in my side ever since. I don't like toaster waffles, yet he insists on making two every morning, as we did that first time. He hands me mine. Big clumps of butter, way too much syrup. Even if we are in a rush, there is no rushing through the morning waffle ritual. I find myself cursing the high fructose corn syrup, the cellulose gum or whatever part of the syrup makes it so slow.

The year previous, breakfasts weren't much better. I was always in a rush. Peter always made an effort to enjoy each bite, savor each mouthful with an

"Mmm" or a "Dat's good" or an "Aah." I set the clock on the stove to beep every thirty seconds to remind Peter it was time to swallow the delicious bite in his mouth and move on to the next, equally satisfying morsel on his plate.

I clumsily orchestrate my four children out the door, maneuver keys, balance a child on my hip. I am on a schedule. It is 8:05 A.M., and I have just three or four minutes to get the kids out of the house and on their way. I make sure little fingers are clear of the hinges, am momentarily preoccupied as the last child lets go of the storm door, which tries every morning to pin me against the front door. Peter, Maggie, Bernadette, baby Bridget and I traverse the steps of our porch together, and then they are gone. I move the baby off my hip and down to the sidewalk, hold her hand as I walk and watch as my kids stretch out before me, along the sidewalk to the corner, where the oldest two will be picked up for school. I watch Maggie's long limbs and graceful strides as she bounds ahead of her brother, Peter running to catch up, hands straight down to his sides. The flats of his feet hit the sidewalk, *thump, thump, thump,* in contrast to Maggie's light *tap, tap, tap,* barely audible. The kids consider the trip to the corner bus stop the day's first treat. I am thinking about the cold, my hands, how I thought I'd served my miserable time waiting for a bus. I am not smiling. The baby and I are two houses behind the others. I cannot see Peter's face, but I know he is smiling and excited. Maggie arrives first at the corner, then Bernadette, finally Peter. I cannot hear what they say, but I see how they chatter, gather closely, laugh.

I arrive and wait with the other neighborhood kids, try to make small talk. I ask a neighborhood girl how her cello lessons are going as I stamp my feet to keep them warm. The bus rounds the corner, and here we say our good-byes for the day. The neighborhood's five riders enter. I watch Maggie make her way back, find a seat, wave. The doors close. I see my reflection in the door windows. I look cold; so does the baby on my hip. Bernadette, only three, stands by my side. She is too young yet for the bus. Peter, my seven-year-old kindergartener/first-grader (spending half the day in each) stands next to me. I remember the Pied Piper and the boy with the crutch, and the memory stings. There is a rawness in this moment as we all look at ourselves reflected in the glass of a bus door. I remind myself that I am too sensitive.

The bus pulls away, and immediately behind it is Peter's bus, a mini, the special-ed bus. Up he goes. A kiss, a hug, and he is gone, waving enthusiastically. I turn and walk back home with the girls, and I think about how, when Peter's bus occasionally arrives first, the kids yell, "The baby bus! The baby bus!" I wonder if they mean that the bus is small or that it is for babies.

It is chaos at our house. We don't always realize it, but the bewildered look on the faces of those who leave—say, after spending an evening—gives it away. It is our family's utterly uncultured and unmannered easiness that is the difficulty. Philip J. Bailey once said, "Lowliness is the base of every virtue, and he who goes the lowest builds the safest." We go for lowliness and have a great time doing it. The kids perform for us. Each has picked a stage name: Christina Arena, Christina Sparkles and Peter Music. We listen as they improvise songs, try out their muses. The Christinas generally sing of love and shoes and the alphabet, with lots of "Oh, yeahs" and "Uh-huhs" throughout. Peter's repertoire is nothing but food. He sings of hot dogs, pizza, McDonalds, ham sandwiches, Sonic, various meats, oatmeal, Burger King, toaster waffles. We're terribly tacky and find these renditions extremely humorous. In addition to being a great lover of food, he is an early riser. More than once I have stumbled out of bed and down the steps to find the entire contents of the refrigerator on the kitchen counter. Living in this house is not always peaceful, but it is often a joy.

Maggie recently told me that she couldn't wait to have another year of kindergarten. I told her that next year she will go to first grade. She asked me why "Peter got two kindergartens." She was right; Peter attended kindergarten the year before, as well. I sat down with her to find out just what she understood. We have explained to her about Down syndrome, and in her understanding, it has a large part to do with Peter's glasses, why he wears them and why she doesn't. I asked her what Down syndrome meant, and she said, "Peter can't do some things so good. He can't see so good, so he wears glasses. But he is the same inside. He has a heart and all that other stuff." I asked her what she thought about Down syndrome, and she responded, "I think it's great. Next question, please."

My favorite part of the annual meeting is the awards banquet, where *consumers* (the word we now use for the people with developmental disabilities that TARC serves) receive awards for their hard work during the previous year. It begins with a group that have agreed to entertain us with their music. They mount the stage via the handicap ramp and proceed to simulate a rainstorm on huge, flat, pielike percussion instruments. They begin by running their hands around and around the circumference of the instrument; it sounds like wind. Next they tap the instruments with their fingers, lightly, lightly, then harder until it really does sound like dozens of raindrops hitting a window or sidewalk. They are then given their drumsticks, foot-long pieces of wood with padded ends. It is then clear why the drumsticks were kept out of their reach. They laugh, shriek with delight, and bang on the drums, bang and bang to simulate thunder.

After the performance I watch as an award for perseverance is given to a man who has worked in the governor's office for more than eight years. He wears a suit jacket, tie, sneakers. He receives his award, searches numerous pockets, and finally pulls out a piece of paper—folded exactly twice—and reads his acceptance speech. "If you work hard, your life will be a success." The paper is refolded and restored to its pocket. He returns to his seat.

The award for enthusiasm is next. The presenter doesn't make it through the introduction before the recipient, a man in his forties, bounds his way to the stage and puts an arm around her. She tries to continue but is repeatedly interrupted by his pleased acclamations of "Whew!" and "This is big!" and "This is real big!" She tries once more to continue and is again interrupted. He yells and points, "There's my mom and dad! Hello Mom and Dad!" Two tiny, old people sitting at a back table smile and wave toward the stage. He shakes his head, is so genuinely pleased. I applaud until my hands itch.

I think about all that we lost that day, and of all that we gained, almost eight years ago, when Peter was born. I think about the human spirit, which rallies, which revels in the ability to get past, to get through. I wonder if it was our bravery or our naïveté that sought brothers or sisters for this child. We considered what it would be like to explain to a child why we, who love children and wanted children, chose to have only one. I never wanted to face my child and say, explicitly or not, "We wanted more, but none like you."

Peter is our oldest but will remain the youngest. Each of his sisters will pass him in height, in knowledge, in vocabulary. I cheer for his small victories. He will always be the first who learned to read. Tim and I take great pride in hearing him read complete sentences; he still doesn't speak in them. At bedtime Peter reads to us all, slowly and deliberately, as he points to each word. We sit on the bed, surround Peter with our bodies, and listen as he reads to us.

Once while visiting the school, Tim and I ran into the principal, who began telling us a story about how one day she heard a ruckus in the hallway and found Mrs. Levins, Peter's special-education teacher, and Peter in an argument there. Peter was irate and yelling, "Homework! Want homework!" Mrs. Levins had no book to send home with him that day and was trying to explain, "No, Peter. No homework today." The principal laughed and told us she had never heard the contention put quite that way before. Mrs. Levins tells us that she thinks we have a recreational reader on our hands. The thought thrills me, and I hope one day he will read books I loved as a kid. *Horton Hears a Who?* Perhaps one day "The Pied Piper"?

Charles Buxton, an English physician, visited Down and recorded his impression of the visit in the Surrey Office Records. Buxton called Down the "right man in the right place" and described how children followed him like the Pied Piper, "taking his hand and evincing their unfeigned delight in his presence." I read this and make a mental note to rethink my opinion of the children's tale.

In 1868 Down purchased Normansfield, a "gentleman's residence" with five acres. In time he acquired the other two houses in the development and more land and opened it all to residents with mental and physical disabilities. On this property he and his wife, Mary, created an environment of learning, providing opportunities for education and craftsmanship, worship and entertainment, to as many as 156 residents at a time. Each staff member was required to have "musical or entertaining skills," which were often showcased in Normansfield's elaborate theater. J. Langdon Down continued work with the "feeble-minded" until his death in 1896.

I have seen several of Down's clinical photographs, which have survived and remain the largest collection of clinical photographs in the United States or Britain. No women in nightdresses, no painted handlebar mustaches or rolled-up stockings to the knees. They are pictures of children in beautiful clothes, collars of lace, embroidered hems. They are pictures of men—like my son, Peter, will one day be—wearing button-down waistcoats and ties, cleanly shaven, hair combed, legs crossed in dark, crisp trousers, hands folded in their laps. Like Velazquez portraits, they are full of dignity.

The final award given at the banquet is for the consumer who has held a job for the longest time. She is a dishwasher at a local restaurant, employed there for ten years. She walks to the podium, head down, hands raised over her head in a thumbs-up gesture, shaking them as marathoners do after crossing the finish line. She proceeds to accept her award. "I just wanna thank the Vintage. I love them at the Vintage, and they's always says that when I finish with the pots and pans, they's look just like they's new. And I love them all at the Vintage, and I turned fifty-one in October, and I gonna work for the Vintage until I a hundred years old. And I pray for the Vintage, but what I really wanna do is sing my music all over the world. I really wanna to be a country singer. But I thank you to the Vintage, and I pray for the Vintage every night. Thank you." She walks down the ramp just the way she walked up, head down, hands above her head, shaking her proud fists with victory.

At last year's banquet, a young man fell on his way to the stage. The room gasped. Members of the crowd got out of their seats to help him up. As he was pulled to his feet, I noticed he was still smiling. He brushed off his jacket and trousers and similarly brushed away those who asked if he was all right. He was on his way to the stage, and no fall, no humiliation, no embarrassment, no well-wishers would slow him down. To those of us who sit and observe, these experiences are invaluable. I slow myself down, *retardatio*, and observe. Learn.

I find that people with little notion about Down syndrome say things like "They are all so loving." Generalizations like this are hard for me to take. I don't lump my girls' personalities because they are girls or because they were born without complication. But the thing that irritates me even more is the realization that sometimes generalizations are true. Peter *is* loving, extremely so. I can discipline him, and he holds no grudge. It is the hardest for me to see him, of all my children, cry. I can't wrench a "Sorry" out of Bernadette, but his is given immediately and sincerely. He is there, present in emotion at every second. He hides nothing, except a package of hot dogs now and then under his shirt. He doesn't laugh out of courtesy. He doesn't know when he is being snubbed. He embraces children who remain stiff, roll their eyes, turn their heads, and he loves it. He is raw, and we relish this about him. I try to seek humility, as he shows it to me daily. I wish I could take some of what people throw his way and send it back to them. I wish I didn't have those desires to throw back at all. I wish I made better use of opportunities to teach others.

I think back to when Peter began kindergarten. All the parents and their students were invited to come the night before, to put away supplies and find a spot at a table. Tim and I arrived with Peter. He picked a table and sat. We watched awkwardly as tables began to fill, while Peter sat alone. He got up to explore, and while he was gone, a little girl and her father picked a spot at Peter's table. When he returned, the father apologetically picked up his daughter's supplies and moved elsewhere. It is at these times I hurt, but only for myself. Peter doesn't notice.

Yet I know he will one day. Until then my heart breaks only for me. I wish I had done Peter justice, perhaps explained him in a kind and objective manner to this little girl's father. I wish I could have pulled out a painting by

Mantegna and a picture of Peter in his ghost costume. I would note the simi-larities of the two little boys with almond eyes, wrapped in sheets. I could tell the story of the Pied Piper. I could use the chalkboard to diagram chromo-somes, provide an introduction to genetics. I could illustrate all my thoughts with an elaborate formula that equals Peter, all that he is and all that he is not.

•

Erin Newport *recently completed her master's degree in English at Kansas State University. She lives in Topeka with her husband and four children.*

The Right Thing

Beth Kephart

∾

L ike a secret whispered in the dark, we ask ourselves what we are owed in this chancy, makeshift life of ours. What we have earned. What we deserve. What is decent, humane, essential. We ask ourselves the question when we are well, and more, we ask it when we are not well, when accident or disease has left us vulnerable, dependent. What are our rights now, we ask ourselves. What are we owed when we are sick?

It isn't just a grown-up worry. It is a question that floats to the surface of too many childhoods. I know, because I remember. I know, because I was the original tomboy—the kickball player with the grand-slam foot and the bright blue bruise upon her knee, the reckless daughter who climbed out windows at night to put a fist around a dancing firefly. I know, because I was injured young, and because it changed my life. Changed the way I saw the world. Left me with questions I'm still asking.

At home my favorite place was the backyard swing, which I owned like I was sure I owned most things. I was the queen of swinging; I made it acrobatic art. I was push off, thrust high, arch back, pump. I was point the toes and atomize the sky. Tucked into the corner of my family's mannered yard, the swing faced a thick-barked, fat-limbed tree. It faced the sun and so I closed my eyes as I hurled my slender body through the clouds.

I sang while I swung, the family standards. The "Trouble" song from *The Music Man*, "When You Wish Upon a Star," and *I've got tears in my ears while I lie on my back in my bed while I cry over you . . .* —you know, those songs. It was

"Blowing in the Wind" that I was belting out to no one when a chinked link on the swing chain snapped and sent me soaring. I'd been headed for the sun, but then I was headed for the tree, and then, like an out-of-favor doll, I was flung down to the ground. I could not breathe until I screamed. I got to my knees, but not to my feet, as I could not pull my left arm from the ground. It lay there flattened, like an old kid glove, and I knew in an instant that the bones inside the skin had been crumpled into pieces: feta cheese.

I remember my father driving and my mother sitting beside me in the backseat of their car. I remember how far the hospital seemed and how the streets were eerily empty. It was Memorial Day Sunday; my father sped through every amber light. When we arrived at last at the hospital, I was transferred to the nurses, laid out on a gurney, and wheeled down corridors. I tried to count the ceiling tiles that sped past in a hurry. Soon, I remember thinking. Soon this pain will stop. But when the gurney reached its destination, there was nothing but time, more pain. Nothing to do but lie in that hallway while a ghoulish green crept up my arm. I waited through hunger, through thirst, through a ripening nausea, through figments and through fears that grew hallucinatory. It was close to midnight by the time the surgeon arrived, sand in his hair, from the beach. Close to midnight, and I know that this is true, because I stared up at the corridor clock and watched its hands colliding.

We're just people until we're hurt or sick, and then we're something else: we're patients. We are the scars, we are the fears, we are the way the trauma changed us. Show me the person who has not been reduced by accident or germs or DNA or a short-staffed ER team, and I'll show you science fiction. We all get on our swing and we all open up and sing and then some chain snaps and sends us flying. A car veers into our lane or a gene comes out of hiding or asbestos filters through our lungs or a heart neglects its purpose. We are human—blood and tissue, cell and spark, vulnerable to the consequence and caprice of our fated, borrowed lives. To be alive is to be at risk. To be healthy today is to understand that tomorrow things may not be the same.

And yet our struggles feel unique and our fears are certainly our own, and there are few things more desperate-making than being sick or loving one who is. Pain is not transferable, never adequately conveyed or shared through words. A machine can tell us where a hurt might reside, but it will not quantify its size. A throb, an ache, an asphyxiating squeeze. A crick, a cramp, a cyst, the collywobbles. Hypopraxia, paroxysm, arrhythmia, pyrexia, tumescence, tumor, crumpled wrist. Tell me yours, I'll tell you mine. We may suffer together, but we never entirely suffer *for* each other. Illness. Injury. Birth defect. Following the diagnoses and the treatment plans, the prescriptions and the rehab, we lie on the raft of our own bodies: prone, alone.

After my surgeon finally arrived that night so long ago, things didn't get better for the nine-year-old with the wrist of feta cheese. I was propped in a chair and put to sleep; I woke up vomiting, in outrageous pain. I woke with my arm in a cast from fingertips to shoulder, and I felt not one whit better or more secure. The cast was stuffed with cotton and it itched like hell and it was destined to get worse throughout the summer. But that didn't matter. What mattered more was this: I knew that despite everything I'd just gone through, my wrist was not healing.

It would be months before the surgeon sawed off that cast and stretched my arm straight and acknowledged what I'd intuited for myself. Months before I was proven right about the body that I lived in. Like an errant iceberg, the head of my ulna was floating free, along the shaft of my arm, and there was nothing to be done, not then; I'd have to wait until my skeleton was fully formed to have the chunk cut loose. I'd spend the next seven years in half-casts and mummy Ace apparel. I'd skate in them and bike in them and try not to look so clubby. And whenever the teachers announced a team sports day in gym (and I hardly remember a day when they didn't) I'd be sent by myself to the library where I, the former tomboy, would sit stock still among the books while my classmates with the stable bones fought hard and unfettered.

We know what happens—what *should* happen—when accident or illness strikes. We know about the mothers with their chicken soup, the sisters at the bedsides, the church elders with the fruit baskets, the fraternity brothers who dial up old friends to give them hope, maybe a cause to laugh, while they await a diagnosis. We know about compassion, empathy, imagination, listening, about cool rags and ice chips, about fresh bouquets and ornaments left inside the mailbox. We know about caring—one for the other—and we also know what the experts say about caring for ourselves, about our responsibility—our right—to stay as healthy as we can: to lower cholesterol, to eat the right things, to not drink and drive, to steer clear of toxins, to submit to checkups, to banish bad habits, to stay off the swings with chinked chains. We have the right to care for those we love, and we have the right to care for ourselves, and we have the right to hope that those who know us will want to care for us.

But that isn't the issue when it comes to patient rights. The issue there, most bluntly put, concerns the rights due us from those doctors, nurses, orderlies, technicians, therapists paid to see us through—from perfect strangers, much of the time, who must prematurely leave their beach house on a holiday weekend to attend to a suddenly smashed-up girl. What are our rights, within the established system? What are our rights, when it comes to the professionals, to insurance carriers and institutions, and to the government? What are our rights, both technically and technologically, in this, our own spectacular era of X-rays and MRIs, antibiotics and radiation, organ donors and plastic hearts, ventilators and IV lines, pharmaceuticals and gene splicing, test-tube babies and thriving preemies, artificial eyes, transplanted hands, implicit promises, surprises? We are patients, we've been patients, we know patients, we'll be patients. And so, we want to know, *What are our rights?*

We are the victims of our own medical knowledge, our own miracle-saturated TV. If one man can replace part of his own missing arm with the actual flesh and bone of another man's arm, why can't anyone struggling with prostheses do the same? If a woman predisposed to early-onset Alzheimer's can save her baby from her genetic fate, why aren't we all given the choice to save children from our own worst traits? If some are saved from the clutches of death with a brand-new heart, shouldn't that option be open to all?

And shouldn't everyone, everywhere, be guaranteed the same quality and attentiveness of care? If I, for example, a young, married woman, am scheduled for surgery to correct a malfunctioning jaw (and I was young once, and this story's true)—if it's planned for, on the books, sanctioned by my insurance carrier, if it comes, in other words, as no shock to anyone—why do I still almost drown in my own blood afterwards, hooked up to a stomach-pumping machine that had already been identified as clogged up, useless, broken? Why do I almost drown? Why do I, with my mouth wired shut, with my arms hooked to machines, with my body wrecked from eight hours of anesthesia, lie helpless in that hospital bed with my blood spitting and arcing all over me, my mind slipping backwards over time the way they say that dying people's minds can do? It was November, near Thanksgiving. Snow was falling outside the window, and the hospital was short on staff. My husband had gone home, after holding vigil until midnight. With the wires through my jaw and a plastic plug between my teeth, the only way that I could speak was to bang a buzzer near my head, and when the blood first began its regurgitation, I banged that buzzer with all my might.

I was not heeded. I watched the crack of light under the hospital-room door, desperate to see shadows, the white hush-hush shoes of nurses. Nothing. Concern grew into disbelief and disbelief into anger and anger into abject fear, and then I just gave up. I was dying. I understood this. I was drowning in my own blood, not from an accident, but from the simple, stupid, mean, and murderous malfunctioning of a machine. I was twenty-six years old. I had not had the child I had intended to have. I had not told my husband good-bye. I had not written a word of the books that I'd known I'd write since I was a child exiled to libraries at the age of nine. I lay back against the red, wet pillow and closed my eyes and died.

Who raised me from the dead was not the nurses, not the doctors, but the stranger in the bed beside me—a beat-up, tough-talking, bar-working gal from West Philadelphia, who'd had the teeth pummeled out of her mouth the night before. It was she who heard me pounding the buzzer, she who woke and came to my bed. She who fixed the damned machine and did not leave my side until morning. Every time the machine got clogged, she cleaned it out. Every time the blood ran down my neck she dabbed it away with a towel. We were, both of us, soaked in my blood by morning. We were, both of us, emotionally wrecked and spiritually bonded, when my husband finally came. We, both of us, gave the nurses attitude when they arrived, with the dawn light, to check their patients. The buzzer, it seemed, had been broken like the pump. Without the perfect stranger from West Philadelphia, I would not be around to tell this story.

Is that right, and is that fair?

Here is what we all know and what we cannot afford to say out loud when we are injured, broken, troubled, or when those we love are, either: Morality, goodness, justice, common sense have no shot at being codified, enacted, enforced so long as humans run this planet. Kindness cannot be legislated. Wisdom is not a single thing. Medicine is bigger than our capacity to wield it. Words can't save us from our own vulnerability, nor can a single bill of patient rights.

And that's because you won't likely find the word *kindness* in most run-of-the-mill bills of patient rights. You won't likely encounter *morality* or *goodness* or *common sense* either. That's not what the laws are all about. Listen to the language of those who devise and dole out patient rights. Listen to those who seek to explain what others have devised and doled out. The Health Law Department of Boston University School of Public Health will be, perhaps, your most helpful guide as you seek to navigate this somewhat nebulous terrain. All medical care, you'll discover, is essentially your choice—which means, in simplest, undogmatic terms, that, first and foremost, you have the right to accept or reject the care you need, and you also have the right not to be trial-and-error monkeyed. Second and further, those to whom you have entrusted your health are, in most patients' bills of rights, legally obligated to provide information: the diagnostic root of the problem, the medical alternatives and attendant consequences, the existence and nature of any experimental treatments, the doctor's honest recommendations, a copy of medical records, a breakdown of medical costs and payment options, a phone number to support the inevitable arbitration. Third, you have the right to bring a family member or friend—a clear-eyed advocate—to any consultation.

Fourth, you have the right to privacy. Fifth, you have the right to not be discriminated against. Sixth, you have the right to refuse to sign any patient consent forms.

There is no cozy language here. There is no one promising to make the migraines a memory, the cancer a has-been, the bad heart able to pump like new, the kidney free of future stones, the salvaged lung capable of inhaling enough for two, the chronic pain remote. No one promising a decent hospital meal or a philosophical roommate or a pretty waiting room or a gracious nurse or an intern who shows up on time. No one even promising that what you "choose" will get paid for in the end—your health, your life, your comfort, your future are worth no more than the Diagnostic Related Groups manual and insurance carrier say they're worth, plus whatever you can dig out of your savings. Patient rights: in many states and hospitals, it signifies no more than the right to information. The right to involve yourself—or is it implicate yourself?—in the choices that are made, which should not be misconstrued as the right to demand an ideal outcome, a humane process, any care beyond the care for which you and your insurer can ultimately pay.

And yet. The system—even today, in the absence of a single standard bill of patient rights—can and does rise to the occasion more than the critics like to say. It does and can heal, it does and can nurture, it does and can revive. Maybe you can't codify rights or legislate the right thing, but you can spot it coming down the hall on quickening shoes. I saw the right thing the night my son was born. I saw it in the technician who worried over my mammogram and in the doctor who treated me late one dinner hour, when I could no longer endure a migraine's pain. I may not believe that words can dictate either right or rights when it comes to patients, but I believe that right gets done. Now and then, or even more than that. I don't have the statistics. I have experience, a feeling.

Or I have, I mean to say, a brother-in-law. A brother-in-law and an indelible memory of the Christmas season, eight years ago, when he very nearly died, was in fact *supposed* to die, and would have, had it not been for the care,

the ingenuity, the love, the determination of an overburdened county hospital. He'd been found by his friends in a pool of his own vomit on the floor in
his apartment, after he'd failed to show for work. He'd been rushed unconscious, unresponsive, to that Dallas institution, where the emergency room
team, empathetic in the crisis of that moment, suspected meningitis, pumped
his body full of antibiotics, and sent him on an urgent gurney to the specialists in intensive care. No waiting. No questions. No red tape. No fuss that he
wasn't, at that time, insured. He was a human being, an absolute stranger,
they knew nothing of his soul, and yet they wanted him to live, and so they
took him under wing, and they settled him into his bed, his machines, and
called on everything they knew and had to help him through the crisis.

My husband caught the first plane out to Dallas and called me that afternoon from a hospital phone. Only a 40 percent chance of survival, he said. If
he lives, he'll be brain-damaged, maybe deaf. And his body is covered with
tremendous fevered boils, as if he had been burned from the inside out. My
husband's brother was deep inside a coma, and his whole body was a fester-
ing wound, and no one knew if he could hear or dream. But from around the
world his family gathered around his bed, his best friends stood, and in the
intensive care unit they weren't giving up, they were fighting for his sake,
determined.

The longer my brother-in-law stayed suspended in that coma, the worse
grew his chances for survival. One day followed another day. Christmas came
and went. Carols were sung in corridors. Small, easing pleasantries were
extended to the family. Each day my husband went and sat beside his brother.
Each day he watched the nurses and the doctors and the interns come and go,
change the dressings, check the machines, resupply the oxygen, lubricate
those swollen lips, that ravaged skin. Christmas and then New Year's, and
then another week went by, and there my brother-in-law lay—an uninsured
man with a less-than-promising prognosis in an intensive care unit in a county
hospital. You see the worst cases here, my husband would call at midnight
and say. You see accidents like you've never seen, all these unimaginable
things. But my brother-in-law was treated with conviction, knowledge,
hope—treated as if he were the only patient among so many imperiled

patients, as if the staff were certain that, despite the odds, he would survive, which he, answering their faith in him, eventually did—the fever leaving its fiery scars, his mind and hearing and soul and heart all, like a TV miracle, strong.

What do we want, when we become patients? We want, first of all, to be understood and to understand. We want the benefit of our era's medical know-how, of the machines that were built and oiled for rescue, of the diagnostic tools. We want not to be diminished even as our bodies fight against us; we want our dignity among the needles and the bedpans. We want to share in what's decided and not be ruined by the costs; we want the care to be humane. We want, above all else, to believe that the right things were done for all the right reasons, at the right place and at the right time. Show me a bill of rights that can guarantee all this, every time, for each and every patient, within any health-care setting, and I'll show you science fiction. Ask me if it's possible, and I'll show you a county hospital in Dallas.

•

Beth Kephart *is the award-winning author of three memoirs. Her third,* Still Love in Strange Places, *about love and loss on a Salvadoran coffee farm, was published in June 2003 by W.W. Norton.*

A Measure of Acceptance

Floyd Skloot
∾

The psychiatrist's office was in a run-down industrial section at the northern edge of Oregon's capital, Salem. It shared space with a chiropractic health center, separated from it by a temporary divider that wobbled in the current created by opening the door. When I arrived a man sitting with his gaze trained on the spot I suddenly filled began kneading his left knee, his suit pants hopelessly wrinkled in that one spot. Another man, standing beside the door and dressed in overalls, studied the empty wall and muttered as he slowly rose on his toes and sank back on his heels. Like me, neither seemed happy to be visiting Dr. Peter Avilov.

Dr. Avilov specialized in the psychodiagnostic examination of disability claimants for the Social Security Administration. He made a career of weeding out hypochondriacs, malingerers, fakers, people who were ill without organic causes. There may be many such scam artists working the disability angle, but there are also many legitimate claimants. Avilov worked as a kind of hired gun, paid by an agency whose financial interests were best served when he determined that claimants were not disabled. It was like having your house appraised by the father-in-law of your prospective buyer, like being stopped by a traffic cop several tickets shy of his monthly quota, like facing a part-time judge who works for the construction company you're suing. Avilov's incentives were not encouraging to me.

I understood why I was there. After a virus I contracted in December of 1988 targeted my brain, I became totally disabled. When the Social Security Administration decided to reevaluate my medical condition eight years later, it exercised its right to send me to a doctor of its own choosing. This seemed fair enough. But after receiving records, test results and reports of brain scans and statements from my own internal-medicine and infectious-diseases physicians, all attesting to my ongoing disability, and after requiring twenty-five pages of handwritten questionnaire answers from me and my wife, the SSA scheduled an appointment for me with Avilov. Not with an independent internal-medicine or infectious-diseases specialist, not with a neurologist, but with a shrink.

Now, twelve years after first getting sick, I've become adept at being brain-damaged. It's not that my symptoms have gone away; I still try to dice a stalk of celery with a carrot instead of a knife, still reverse "p" and "b" when I write, or draw a primitive hourglass when I mean to draw a star. I call our *bird feeder* a *breadwinner* and place newly purchased packages of frozen corn in the dishwasher instead of the freezer. I put crumpled newspaper and dry pine into our wood stove, strike a match, and attempt to light the metal door. Preparing to cross the "main street" in Carlton, Oregon, I look both ways, see a pickup truck a quarter-mile south, take one step off the curb, and land flat on my face, cane pointing due east.

So I'm still much as I was in December of 1988, when I first got sick. I spent most of a year confined to bed. I couldn't write and had trouble reading anything more complicated than *People* magazine or the newspaper's sports page. The functioning of memory was shattered, bits of the past clumped like a partly assembled jigsaw puzzle, the present a flicker of discontinuous images. Without memory it was impossible for me to learn how to operate the new music system that was meant to help me pass the time, or figure out why I felt so confused, or take my medications without support.

But in time I learned to manage my encounters with the world in new ways. I shed what no longer fit my life: training shoes and road-racing flats,

three-piece suits and ties, a car. I bought a cane. I seeded my home with pads
and pens so that I could write reminders before forgetting what I'd thought.
I festooned my room with color-coded Post-It notes telling me what to do,
whom to call, where to locate important items. I remarried, finding love when
I imagined it no longer possible. Eventually I moved to the country, slowing
my external life to match its internal pace, simplifying, stripping away layers
of distraction and demands.

Expecting the unexpected now, I can, like an improvisational actor,
incorporate it into my performance. For instance, my tendency to use words
that are close to—but not exactly—the words I'm trying to say has led to
some surprising discoveries in the composition of sentences. A freshness
emerges when the mind is unshackled from its habitual ways. In the past I
never would have described the effect of a viral attack on my brain as being
"geezered" overnight if I hadn't first confused the words *seizure* and *geezer.* It
is as though my word-finding capacity has developed an associative function
to compensate for its failures of precision, so I end up with *shellac* instead of
plaque when trying to describe the gunk on my teeth. Who knows, maybe
James Joyce was brain-damaged when he wrote *Finnegan's Wake* and built a
whole novel on puns and neologisms that were actually symptoms of disease.

It's possible to see such domination of the unexpected in a positive light.
So getting lost in the familiar woods around our house and finding my way
home again add a twist of excitement to days that might seem circumscribed
or routine because of my disability. When the natural-food grocery where we
shop rearranged its entire stock, I was one of the few customers who didn't
mind, since I could never remember where things were anyway. I am less
hurried and more deliberate than I was; being attentive, purposeful in movement, lends my life an intensity of awareness that was not always present
before. My senses are heightened, their fine-tuning mechanism busted. Spicy
food, stargazer lilies in bloom, birdsong, heat, my wife's vivid palette when
she paints—all have become more intense and stimulating. Because it threatens my balance, a sudden breeze is something to stop for, to let its strength
and motion register. That may not guarantee success—as my pratfall in Carlton indicates—but it does allow me to appreciate detail and nuance.

One way of spinning this is to say that my daily experience is often spontaneous and exciting. Not fragmented and intimidating, but unpredictable, continuously new. I may lose track of things, or of myself in space, my line of thought, but instead of getting frustrated, I try to see this as the perfect time to stop and figure out what I want or where I am. I accept my role in the harlequinade. It's not so much a matter of making lemonade out of life's lemons but rather of learning to savor the shock, taste, texture and aftereffects of a mouthful of unadulterated citrus.

Acceptance is a deceptive word. It suggests compliance, a consenting to my condition and to who I have become. This form of acceptance is often seen as weakness, submission. We say, *I accept my punishment.* Or *I accept your decision.* But such assent, while passive in essence, does provide the stable, rocklike foundation for coping with a condition that will not go away. It is a powerful passivity, the Zen of Illness, that allows for endurance.

There is, however, more than endurance at stake. A year in bed, another year spent primarily in my recliner—these were times when endurance was the main issue. But over time I began to recognize the possibilities for transformation. I saw another kind of acceptance as being viable, the kind espoused by Robert Frost when he said, "Take what is given, and make it over your own way." That is, after all, the root meaning of the verb "to accept," which comes from the Latin *accipere,* or "to take to oneself." It implies an embrace. Not a giving up but a welcoming. People encourage the sick to resist, to fight back; we say that our resistance is down when we contract a virus. But it wasn't possible to resist the effects of brain damage. Fighting to speak rapidly and clearly, as I always had in the past, only leads to more garbling of meaning; willing myself to walk without a cane or climb a ladder only leads to more falls; demanding that I not forget something only makes me angrier when all I can remember is the effort not to forget. I began to realize that the most aggressive act I could perform on my own behalf was to stop struggling and discover what I really could do.

This, I believe, is what the Austrian psychotherapist Viktor E. Frankl refers to in his classic book, *The Doctor and the Soul*, as "spiritual elasticity." He says, speaking of his severely damaged patients, "Man must cultivate the flexibility to swing over to another value-group if that group and that alone offers the possibility of actualizing values." Man must, Frankl believes, "temper his efforts to the chances that are offered."

Such shifts of value, made possible by active acceptance of life as it is, can only be achieved alone. Doctors, therapists, rehabilitation professionals, family members, friends, lovers cannot reconcile a person to the changes wrought by illness or injury, though they can ease the way. Acceptance is a private act, achieved gradually and with little outward evidence. It also seems never to be complete; I still get furious with myself for forgetting what I'm trying to tell my daughter during a phone call, humiliated when I blithely walk away with another shopper's cart of groceries or fall in someone's path while examining the lower shelves at Powell's Bookstore.

But for all its private essence, acceptance cannot be expressed purely in private terms. My experience did not happen to me alone; family, colleagues and friends, acquaintances all were involved. I had a new relationship with my employer and its insurance company, with federal and state government, with people who read my work. There is a social dimension to the experience of illness and to its acceptance, a kind of reciprocity between self and world that goes beyond the enactment of laws governing handicapped access to buildings or rules prohibiting discrimination in the workplace. It is in this social dimension that, for all my private adjustment, I remain a grave cripple and, apparently, a figure of contempt.

At least the parties involved agreed that what was wrong with me was all in my head. However, mine was disability arising from organic damage to the brain caused by a viral attack, not from psychiatric illness. The distinction matters; my disability status would not continue if my condition were psychiatric. It was in the best interests of the Social Security Administration for Dr.

Avilov to say my symptoms were caused by the mind, were psychosomatic rather than organic in nature. And what was in their interests was also in Avilov's.

On high-tech scans, tiny holes in my brain make visually apparent what is clear enough to anyone who observes me in action over time: I no longer have "brains." A brain, yes, with many functions intact, but I'm not as smart or as quick or as steady as I was. Though I may not look sick, and I don't shake or froth or talk to myself, after a few minutes it becomes clear that something fundamental is wrong. My losses of cognitive capability have been fully measured and recorded. They were used by the Social Security Administration and the insurance company to establish my total disability, by various physicians to establish treatment and therapy programs, by a pharmaceutical company to establish my eligibility for participation in the clinical field trial of a drug that didn't work. I have a handicapped parking placard on the dashboard of my car; I can get a free return-trip token from the New York City subway system by flashing my Medicaid card. In this sense I have a public profile as someone who is disabled. I have met the requirements.

Further, as someone with quantifiable diminishment in IQ levels, impaired abstract reasoning and learning facility, scattered recall capacities and aptitudes which decrease as fatigue or distraction increases, I am of scientific use. When it serves their purposes, various institutions welcome me. Indeed they pursue me. I have been actively recruited for three experimental protocols run by Oregon Health Sciences University. One of these, a series of treatments using DMSO, made me smell so rancid that I turned heads just by walking into a room. But when it does not serve their purpose, these same institutions dismiss me. Or challenge me. No matter how well I may have adjusted to living with brain damage, the world I often deal with has not. When money or status is involved, I am positioned as a pariah.

So would Avilov find that my disability was continuing, or would he judge me as suffering from mental illness? Those who say that the distinction is bogus, or that the patient's fear of being labeled mentally ill is merely a cultural bias and ought not matter, are missing the point. Money is at stake; in our culture this means it matters very much. To all sides.

Avilov began by asking me to recount the history of my illness. He seemed as easily distracted as I was; while I stared at his checked flannel shirt, sweetly ragged mustache and the pen he occasionally put in his mouth like a pipe, Avilov looked from my face to his closed door to his empty notepad and back to my face, nodding. When I finished, he asked a series of diagnostic questions: Did I know what day it was (Hey, I'm here on the right day, aren't I?), could I name the presidents of the United States since Kennedy, could I count backward from one hundred by sevens? During this series he interrupted me to provide a list of four unconnected words (such as *train argue barn vivid*), which I was instructed to remember for later recall. Then he asked me to explain what was meant by the expression "People who live in glass houses should not throw stones." I nodded, thought for a moment, knew that this sort of proverb relied on metaphor, which, since I was a poet, should be my great strength, and began to explain. Except that I couldn't. I must have talked for five minutes, in tortuous circles, spewing gobbledygook about stones breaking glass and people having things to hide, shaking my head, backtracking as I tried to elaborate. But it was beyond me, as all abstract thinking is beyond me, and I soon drifted into stunned silence. Crashing into your limitations this way hurts; I remembered as a long-distance runner hitting the fabled "wall" at about mile 22 of the Chicago Marathon, my body depleted of all energy resources, feeding on its own muscle and fat for every additional step, and I recognized this as being a similar sensation.

For the first time, I saw something clear in Avilov's eyes. He saw me. He recognized this as real, the blathering of a brain-damaged man who still thinks he can think.

It was at this moment that he asked, "Why are you here?"

I nearly burst into tears, knowing that he meant I seemed to be suffering from organic rather than mental illness. Music to my ears. "I have the same question."

The rest of our interview left little impression. But when the time came for me to leave, I stood to shake his hand and realized that Avilov had forgotten to ask me if I remembered the four words I had by then forgotten. I did remember having to remember them, though. Would it be best to walk out of the room, or should I remind him that he forgot to have me repeat the words I could no longer remember? Or had I forgotten that he did ask me, lost as I was in the fog of other failures? Should I say, *I can't remember if you asked me to repeat those words, but there's no need because I can't remember them?*

None of that mattered because Avilov, bless his heart, had found that my disability status remained as it was. Such recommendations arrive as mixed blessings; I would much rather not be as I am, but since I am, I must depend on receiving the legitimate support I paid for when healthy and am entitled to now.

There was little time to feel relieved because I soon faced an altogether different challenge, this time from the company that handled my disability-insurance payments. I was ordered to undergo a two-day "Functional Capacity Evaluation" administered by a rehabilitation firm the insurer hired in Portland. A later phone call informed me to prepare for six and a half hours of physical challenges the first day and three hours more the following day. I would be made to lift weights, carry heavy boxes, push and pull loaded crates, climb stairs, perform various feats of balance and dexterity, complete puzzles, answer a barrage of questions. But I would have an hour for lunch.

Wear loose clothes. Arrive early.

With the letter had come a warning: "You must provide your best effort so that the reported measurements of your functional ability are valid." Again the message seemed clear: No shenanigans, you! We're wise to your kind.

I think the contempt that underlies these confrontations is apparent. The patient, or—in the lingo of insurance operations—the claimant, is approached not only as an adversary but as a deceiver. *You can climb more stairs than that! You really can stand on one leg like a heron! Stop falling over, freeloader! We know that game.* Paranoia rules; here an institution seems caught in its grip. With money at stake, the disabled are automatically supposed to be up to some kind of chicanery, and our displays of symptoms are viewed as untrustworthy. Never mind that I contributed to Social Security for my entire working life, with the mutual understanding that if I were disabled the fund would be there for me. Never mind that both my employer and I paid for disability insurance with the mutual understanding that if I were disabled, payments would be there for me. Our doctors are suspect, our caregivers implicated. *We've got our eyes on you!*

The rehab center looked like a combination gym and children's playground. The staff was friendly, casual. Several were administering physical therapy so that the huge room into which I was led smelled of sweat. An elderly man at a desk worked with a small stack of blocks. Above the blather of Muzak, I heard grunts and moans of pained effort: a woman lying on mats, being helped to bend damaged knees; a stiff-backed man laboring through his stretches; two women side by side on benches, deep in conversation as they curled small weights.

The man assigned to conduct my Functional Capacity Evaluation looked enough like me to be a cousin. Short, bearded, thick hair curling away from a lacy bald spot, Reggie shook my hand and tried to set me at ease. He was good at what he did, lowering the level of confrontation, expressing compassion, concerned about the effect on my health of such strenuous testing. I should let him know if I needed to stop.

Right then, before the action began, I had a moment of grave doubt. I could remain suspicious, paranoia begetting paranoia, or I could trust Reggie to be honest, to assess my capacities without prejudice. The presence of patients being helped all around me seemed a good sign. This firm didn't appear dependent upon referrals for evaluation from insurance companies; it had a lucrative operation independent of all that. And if I could not trust a man who reminded me of a healthier version of myself, it seemed like bad karma. I loved games and physical challenges. But I knew who and what I was now; it would be fine if I simply let him know as well. Besides, he was sharp enough to recognize suspicion in my eyes, anyway, and that would give him reason to doubt my efforts. Though much of my disability results from cognitive deficits, there are physical manifestations, too, so letting Reggie know me in the context of a gymlike setting felt comfortable. We were both after the same thing: a valid representation of my abilities. Now was the time to put all I had learned about acceptance on the line. It would require a measure of acceptance on both sides.

What I was not prepared for was how badly I would perform in every test. I knew my limitations but had never measured them. Over a dozen years, the consequences of exceeding my physical capabilities had been made clear enough that I learned to live within the limits. Here I was brought repeatedly to those limits and beyond. After an hour with Reggie, I was ready to sleep for the entire next month. The experience was crushing. How could I comfortably manage only 25 pounds in the floor-to-waist lift repetitions? I used to press 150 pounds as part of my regular weekly training for competitive racing. How could I not stand on my left foot for more than two seconds? You shoulda seen me on a ball field! I could hold my arms up for no more than seventy-five seconds, could push a cart loaded with no more than 40 pounds of weights, could climb only sixty-six stairs. I could not fit shapes into their proper holes in a form-board in the time allotted, though I distinctly remember playing a game with my son that worked on the same principles and always beating the timer. Just before lunch Reggie asked me to squat and lift a box filled with paper. He stood behind me and was there as I fell back into his arms.

As Dr. Avilov had already attested, I was not clinically depressed, but this evaluation was almost enough to knock me into the deepest despair. Reggie said little to reveal his opinions. At the time, I thought that meant that he was simply being professional, masking judgment, and though I sensed empathy, I realized that could be a matter of projection on my part.

Later I believed that his silence came from knowing what he had still to make me do. After lunch and an interview about the Activities of Daily Living form I had filled out, Reggie led me to a field of blue mats spread across the room's center. For a moment I wondered if he planned to challenge me to a wrestling match. That thought had lovely, symbolic overtones: wrestling with someone who suggested my former self; wrestling with an agent of *them*, a man certain to defeat me; or having my Genesis experience, like Jacob at

Peniel wrestling with Him. Which, at least for Jacob, resulted in a blessing and a nice payout.

But no. Reggie told me to crawl.

In order to obtain "a valid representation" of my abilities, it was necessary for the insurance company to see how far and for how long and with what result I could crawl. It was a test I had not imagined. It was a test which could, in all honesty, have only one purpose. My ability to crawl could not logically be used as a valid measure of my employability. And in light of all the other tasks I had been unable to perform, crawling was not necessary as a measure of my functional limits. It would test nothing, at least nothing specific to my case, not even the lower limits of my capacity. Carrying the malign odor of indifference, tyranny's tainted breath, the demand that I crawl was almost comical in its obviousness: the paternal powers turning someone like me, a disabled man living in dependence upon their finances, into an infant.

I considered refusing to comply. Though the implied threat *(You must provide your best effort . . .)* contained in their letter crossed my mind, and I wondered how Beverly and I would manage without my disability payments, it wasn't practicality that made me proceed. At least I don't think so. It was, instead, acceptance. I had spent the morning in a public confrontation with the fullness of my loss, as though on stage, with Reggie, representing the insurance company, as my audience. Now I would confront the sheer heartlessness of The System, the powers that demanded that I crawl before they agreed temporarily to accept my disability. I would, perhaps for the first time, join the company of those far more damaged than I am, who have endured far more indignity in their quest for acceptance. Whatever it was that Reggie and the insurance company believed they were measuring as I got down on my hands and knees and began a slow circuit of the mats in the center of that huge room, I believed I was measuring how far we still had to go for acceptance.

Reggie stood in the center of the mats, rotating in place as I crawled along one side, turned at the corner, crossed to the opposite side, and began to return toward the point where I had started. Before I reached it, Reggie told me to stop. He had seen enough. I was slow and unsteady at the turns, but I could crawl fine.

I never received a follow-up letter from the insurance company. I was never formally informed of its findings, though my disability payments have continued.

At the end of the second day of testing, Reggie told me how I'd done. In many of the tests, my results were in the lowest 5–10 percent for men my age. My performance diminished alarmingly on the second day, and he hadn't ever tested anyone who did as poorly on the dexterity components. He believed that I had given my best efforts and would report accordingly. But he would not give me any formal results. I was to contact my physician, who would receive Reggie's report in due time.

When the battery of tests had first been scheduled, I'd made an appointment to see my doctor a few days after their completion. I knew the physical challenges would worsen my symptoms and wanted him to see what had resulted. I knew I would need his help. By the time I got there, he too had spoken to Reggie and knew about my performance. But my doctor never got an official report, either.

This was familiar ground. Did I wish to request a report? I was continuing to receive my legitimate payments; did I really want to contact my insurance company and demand to see the findings of my Functional Capacity Evaluation? Risk waking the sleeping dragon? What would be the point? I anticipated no satisfaction in reading that I was in fact disabled or in seeing how my experience translated into numbers or bureaucratic prose.

It seems that I was only of interest when there was an occasion to rule me ineligible for benefits. Found again to be disabled, I wasn't even due the courtesy of a reply. The checks came; what more did I need to show that my claims were accepted?

There was no need for a report. Through the experience, I had discovered something more vital than the measures of my physical capacity. The measure of public acceptance that I hoped to find, that I imagined would balance my private acceptance, was not going to come from a public agency or public corporation. It didn't work that way, after all. The public was largely indifferent, as most people, healthy or not, understand. The only measure of acceptance would come from how I conducted myself in public, moment by moment. With laws in place to permit handicapped access to public spaces, prevent discrimination, and encourage involvement in public life, there is general acceptance that the handicapped live among us and must be accommodated. But that doesn't mean they're not resented, feared, or mistrusted by the healthy. The Disability Racket!

I had encountered the true, hard heart of the matter. My life in the social dimension of illness is governed by forces that are severe and implacable. Though activism has helped protect the handicapped over the last four decades, there is little room for reciprocity between the handicapped person and his or her world. It is naive to expect otherwise.

I would like to think that the insurance company didn't send an official letter of findings because it was abashed at what it had put me through. I would like to think that Dr. Avilov, who no longer practices in Salem, hasn't moved away because he found too many claimants disabled and lost his contract with the Social Security Administration. That my experience educated Reggie and his firm and that his report educated the insurance company, so everyone now understands the experience of disability or of living with brain damage.

But I know better. My desire for reciprocity between self and world must find its form in writing about my experience. Slowly. This essay has taken me eleven months to complete, in sittings of fifteen minutes or so. Built of fragments shaped after the pieces were examined, its errors of spelling and of word choice and logic ferreted out with the help of my wife or daughter or computer's spell-checker. It may look to a reader like the product of someone a lot less damaged than I claim to be. But it's not. It's the product of someone who has learned how to live with his limitations and work with them. And when it's published, if someone employed by my insurance company reads it, I will probably get a letter in the mail demanding that I report for another battery of tests. After all, this is not how a brain-damaged man is supposed to behave.

•

Floyd Skloot, author of the recent memoir In the Shadow of Memory, *is a poet, novelist, and essayist whose work has appeared in such distinguished American magazines as* The Atlantic Monthly, Harper's, Poetry, The American Scholar, Utne Reader, Georgia Review, Boulevard, Shenandoah, Sewanee Review, *and* Southern Review. *Skloot's work has appeared in the* Pushcart Prize Anthology 2004, The Best American Science Writing 2000 *and* 2003, *and* The Best American Essays 1993 *and* 2000.

Rachel at Work

Enclosed, a Mother's Report

Jane Bernstein

∿

In the spring of 2002, as the crocuses pushed up and the daffodils blossomed and froze, I worried about work—not my own, which I love, but what kind of work my developmentally disabled eighteen-year-old daughter Rachel might be able to do when she is no longer in the shelter of school.

On one April morning—an average morning, in fact—after quarreling with her because she would not put her dishes in the dishwasher and threatening to take away her Uno cards if she did not brush her teeth, I asked her if she knew what *work* meant. After a few false starts—trying to make a case for computer solitaire as work, for instance—she pretty much nailed it. Work, she said, was "when you have to do stuff they ask you to do."

Did she like to work? I asked.

"Not really."

"How come?"

"'Cause the way they talk to me is really mean. They talk harsh on me, Ma. Put it this way: When they talk to me, they tell me to be quiet and all that junk."

Outside, a horn honked. I trailed behind Rachel as she reached for the banister and slowly edged her way down the porch steps, then into the van that takes her to the Children's Institute, where, on a typical day, she will sort and deliver mail, make a bed, and wipe down a table.

After the van pulled away from the sidewalk, I stood for a moment, limp from a combination of exhaustion and relief, since my daughter, with her long list of "special needs," is an exceedingly difficult person, especially in the morning and evening when I ask her to do the routines that most of us do without much thought. Most of us—*us* meaning the population that designates itself "normal"—don't need to be prompted to use the toilet, don't at eighteen insist on wearing a sweat suit on a day when the temperature might reach eighty. We don't finish breakfast with a ring of food around our mouths—or if we do, are grateful when someone says, "Honey, you've got food on your face." Most of us don't mind touching our own faces to wipe the food off. While often I am reminded that Rachel is one of us, deserving of the rights and privileges accorded to her by our constitution, on this morning— during this whole season, while I have been thinking about how to make her into a working girl—I have been reminded instead of all the impediments in her way.

I always imagined that Rachel would work. Even after it became obvious that she would never read books or write a single sentence, after I realized that she would never walk on the street alone or live without supervision, I had a vision of her having some sort of job, somewhere. When I saw a janitor or a person busing tables, I would close my eyes and try to picture Rachel doing that job, sure that despite her cognitive deficits, her poor vision and poor fine-motor skills, she could be trained for some job, somewhere. I speculated on the challenges of making a worker out of someone like my daughter, who is unable to understand concepts like altruism and loyalty, who doesn't seem to take pleasure from a job well done and would never fear being fired. Still I went to sleep at night believing that some job would be found and that the structure and routine it provided would be good for her. Unlike many of *us*, her capacity for happiness was great, it seemed. All we had to do was help her find a job and a safe place to live, and we would be on our way.

My vague dream was nourished by several factors: First, that Rachel would be in school until she was nearly twenty-two. Second, that she had been given an after-school job at Café J, a snack bar staffed by people with special needs at the Jewish Community Center near our home. Though a trained therapeutic staff-support person (TSS) was always at her side, making sure her behavior was appropriate and keeping her on task, still it was work. Third, I believed in some equally vague way that the law would protect her. In the back of my mind was the knowledge that if Rachel had been born less than a generation ago, I would have been advised—pressured, perhaps—to put her into an institution. Even if I had ample funds, I would have been hard-pressed to find a nearby school she could attend. In those days a conversation with the words *work* and *Rachel* in the same sentence would not have been even vaguely feasible. The Developmental Disabilities Assistance and Bill of Rights Act of 1975 and the Education for All Handicapped Children Act of 1975 (now called Individuals with Disabilities Education Act, or IDEA) passed only eight years before Rachel's birth. They guaranteed her access to free education, the chance to find decent, affordable housing in her own community, the opportunity to work and play—in short, the right to choose how and where she wanted to live.

I was lulled by these laws and by the fact that thus far I had not had to fight for Rachel's right to be educated. In New Jersey, where we had lived until she was eight, she'd had excellent services, starting with an early-intervention program she attended as an infant. And when I moved to Pittsburgh, ready to fight if necessary to have her placed in an approved private school of my choosing, the school district looked at her medical and educational documents from New Jersey and cooperated fully with my desires. In 1992 she began attending the Children's Institute, and since then the school has been fulfilling the law by providing her education.

When Rachel turned fourteen, she began the "transition process" as stipulated by a 1997 revision of IDEA, the time when we—parents, educators and Rachel herself—were supposed to begin to prepare her for life beyond school. Each summer since then, I'd filled out long questionnaires with dozens of questions about her likes and dislikes. I listed the agencies that had worked with her, the stores and restaurants she liked. I wrote down her favorite foods and games, her after-school activities and some activities I wanted to see her try. Could she be trusted with money? I was asked. Did she understand the passage of time? Could she accept responsibility for her actions, make appointments, talk on the phone? I answered these questions carefully, with her best interests in mind. I prided myself on being realistic, believed that I had no illusions about my expectations for my daughter. I could see the big picture, I would have said.

Then in September 2001, I opened a manila envelope from Rachel's school, looked at her curriculum for that academic year, and saw *washing machine, dryer, setting the table.* I didn't think, *This is great,* or even, *This is the law.* I thought, full of utter despair, *They've given up.* Of course I knew that she'd been working at school — she and her class had tried out some lawn-maintenance jobs and had torn paper for the kennels at the Animal Rescue League — but her educational program in past years had included looking at preprimers, sounding out words, learning to develop a sight vocabulary, answering verbal-comprehension questions about a story, counting by rote to thirty-five, identifying seasonal changes, the needs of a plant, the characteristics of lions, tigers, elephants. Though she continued to function well below grade level, the tone in the mostly boilerplate documents had always been full of strategies that would be employed and accommodations that would be made for her, full of hope for what she might yet become.

The language in the document that set out her plan for the 2001–2002 academic year was blunt: "Due to neurological disabilities and extensive need for modification in all areas, Rachel is unable at this time to participate in the general regular education curriculum." She would be in the Life Skills Program instead. Her goals would be to learn the location of classrooms, sort mail by number up to twenty with 60 percent accuracy, count five items without cues, collate four color-coded items with verbal cues. The tasks seemed so meager — so pathetically small. First I bristled. Then I thought, *She really is retarded,* though for eighteen years I had known this, believed I had accepted it fully. But there was something final about it — *is and always will be* "unable to participate." Looking at this document, I was forced to see that progress for this school year was being measured by my eighteen-year-old daughter's ability to deliver mail independently to a two-room route in a building she had known for nine years.

In October at the meeting to discuss her IEP — Individual Educational Plan — I said I wanted her teachers to continue working with her on some basic academic skills, since I believed it was important for Rachel to know the difference between Women's Room and Men's Room, between Entrance and Exit, Cheerios and Frosted Flakes. And indeed, with just the spirit of coop-eration I'd always felt at these meetings, a few additional goals were drafted: that Rachel would "identify words related to shopping, community signs, menus and recipes," that she would make change up to one dollar. I thanked her teachers and the representative from the school district for working with Rachel and left the building alone.

I was still reeling, utterly stunned. What about the progress she'd been making at the café? Her TSS had been telling me that lately she had been more cooperative about working, that she was using the cash register and closing up the café without being reminded of the sequence of tasks she had to do. Yes, I understood that the JCC café was a protected environment and that she had someone at her side prompting and cueing and redirecting. Still, two rooms without distraction — was that the most her teachers at the Chil-dren's Institute thought she could achieve?

The only way I would learn whether I was deluded or her teachers underestimated her abilities was to observe her in class. But several months would pass before I stepped into her school. And that, I think, had to do with the fourth reason I had held onto my some-job-somewhere dream and let myself imagine that those 1975 laws would be carried out flawlessly, that along with *some* job for Rachel, there would be *someplace* for her to live, some guaranteed safety net. I was tired. Rachel is a difficult person. She gets fund-ing for mental health services because of her "long history of behavior prob-lems, particularly when she is with her mother." Whatever doesn't require my urgent attention goes into an okay-for-the-present category. Her teachers and staff were there, and so had been her future when she was out of school.

I've tried hard to understand my inscrutable daughter. I listen to her, interact with her, worry about her. I've accommodated her deficits and championed her strengths and thought of myself as her advocate and her interpreter, the one who understood her best. That spring, after visiting Rachel's school, I realized that I had failed to integrate all I knew about Rachel. My view of my daughter was limited. So was my understanding of "work."

Here's what I learned.

1. Rachel must learn how to make toast.

She was around five when we started working with her to put on her own shoes. An occupational therapist strung elastic laces in her shoes so that tying and untying would be unnecessary. Then we reinforced—and reinforced—the procedure, starting with "off," which was easier. First you sit in a chair. Next you bring one leg up and over the other. Cross that leg. Reach for the heel of the shoe. Pull. It was the first time I considered how complicated, and how frustrating, it might be to take off one's shoe.

I thought about teaching Rachel to put on her shoes when I observed her morning cooking class. The group had been doing a unit on breakfast, and on this particular morning, their teacher, Bob Russell, produced a bag of bread and announced that the topic for the day was toast. Learning to make toast, like putting on one's shoes, is a multistep operation. First you had to wipe down the counter "because you might drop the toast, and germs are *gross!*" Then you had to figure out what you wanted to put on the toast. And then, after the students slowly offered suggestions for what they might put on their bread—butter, peanut butter, margarine, jam—they had to figure out where they might find these things.

For instance, "Where is butter kept?" Bob asked. What about the jelly?

So you have this purple jelly. What flavor is purple? What flavor is the red?

Sometimes you have to push hard on the handle to get the bread to go down. Sometimes you don't.

How do you get the containers open? Sometimes you lift the lid. Sometimes you unscrew the jar.

What do you use to get the stuff out—a spoon or a knife? Can you manage a butter knife, or will you need a broad, flexible spreader?

Safety. Germs. Hand-washing. Choice. Spreading what you've chosen to go on the toast as evenly as possible. Trying to cut the toast in half.

That night at dinner, I sat across the table from my daughter and heard myself say, "Don't shove giant chunks into your mouth. . . . Chew your food—with your mouth closed please. . . . Use a napkin. . . . Wipe your face and hands."

I thought about work not merely as a specific job or career but as "exertion" and "effort," which also are definitions. I thought of how hard Rachel worked, how for her getting dressed is work. So is clearing the breakfast table, brushing her teeth, negotiating the front steps on a sunny day. Even eating was full of lessons: You could choke. You'll gross people out. Cleanliness counts. Little is self-evident to my daughter, since she is not attuned to matters of safety or health or other people's judgment of her. And these small, necessary things—cutting her food into smaller pieces, opening the napkin, wiping her fingers—are labor for her.

At the same time, she can be astoundingly lazy, capable of standing for a half-hour in the shower and never once reaching for the soap. She tries to manipulate everyone she meets. The instant a new person is within earshot, my princess of Pittsburgh will get that person to lift, tote, fetch, serve and attend to her every need.

Rachel must learn to make her own toast. Even if she is blessed with the most accommodating friend or aide, she must learn to choose what she wants to eat and where she wants to go. She must be responsible for basic hygiene and cleanliness. The more independent she becomes, the better chance she has for being out in the world, something my gregarious daughter craves. The domestic skills she learns will carry her beyond the kitchen into the world where things have levers, lids and screw tops, are stored in cabinets behind wooden doors, where there are slots, stairs, escalators that go up and down, revolving doors. Learning to make toast is helping her live with dignity. Toast is more than toast.

And "life skills" doesn't mean this is the end. They are the necessary skills that will help her be part of a community and part of the working world.

2. Supported employment is not a sure thing.

To most people there's a single face of individuals with mental retardation out there in the workplace: the supermarket bagger. It's the most visible job, the one we see most often. A bagger, like my pal Jimmy, an older man, balding, missing a few teeth, who bags groceries efficiently and carefully at the local supermarket, heavy stuff on the bottom, the eggs in a separate bag. (When Jimmy sees me, he stops, opens his arms wide, grunts with utter glee, and then *pronto* is back to work.) According to the 1990 census, about 87 percent of the 6.2 to 7.5 million people in the United States with mental retardation are, like Jimmy, mildly affected, a little slower than average in learning new information and skills. In the workplace they have proven to be diligent and loyal; they don't job-hop or pose any additional health or safety issues.

At Rachel's school this kind of "competitive employment" is only one of three categories for students in the transition program and a possibility only for those who can become independent, can learn time-management skills, and have the ability to use public transportation—all this before mastering the job itself. Other students are learning skills that will enable them to seek "supported employment," in a sheltered environment. In the third group are those with the most extreme health problems and disabilities, who will go to respite care or an adult training facility.

In April 2002 I visited a work-production class where students were learning specific skills.

When I visited Bob Russell's class, I learned that making toast was more than figuring out how brown you liked your bread. After I visited Dawn Tomlin's class, I understood that succeeding in work production meant not merely mastering specific job skills, like sorting, counting or tallying, but also improving "time-on-task" skills, such as endurance, work rate and speed. Good workers must be able to interact properly with each other. They have to learn to ask for supplies when they run short and seek help if there is something they don't understand.

Dawn's room was wonderfully familiar, on its walls a map of the world, a poster of baseball legend Roberto Clemente, a banner that read, *Understand the similarities. Celebrate the differences.*

The day of my visit, seven students sat around a long table. For several class periods, they'd been helping refurbish science kits for area schools for the Asset Project. The plastic pieces—thousands of them—for these kits had been separated into storage bins and stacked on the shelves of a cart. That afternoon the first job was sorting two tires into a Ziploc bag.

Two students were in wheelchairs. One had partial use of one hand. The other boy, Robin, writhed continuously. On the tray of his wheelchair was a state-of-the-art language board that had been programmed to say at his command the kinds of things any student might need to say, for instance, "I need more supplies." He needed only to touch an icon on the board for it to speak. It was quite forgiving. The board "understood" Robin even when his aim was imperfect.

Five other workers were at the table—two dreamy-looking kids, and three others, including Rachel, on this day wearing her purple shirt and two strands of purple Mardi Gras beads. A teacher, two aides and a student teacher were also helping out.

"Everyone will start with a yellow bin," Dawn said in a loud, clear voice. "Everyone will have—what do you have? A tire. You have to put two tires into one bag. This is the first step. Okay. Does everybody have a large tire? Everybody should have a large tire. Now, what do you need?"

"A bag!" someone eventually offered.

"Set two tires aside. You're going to have to put two—listen, Jake. *Two* tires into *one* bag. Okay? This is the first step."

And so they began, each with his or her spectrum of behavioral, cognitive and physical limitations. Each with issues. In this class, as in cooking, Rachel's were less apparent. My being at her school had put her into a bashful mode.

The boys in the wheelchairs first worked the tires into a plastic container.

This made it easier for them to slide the tires into the Ziploc bag. If the sheer effort was obvious, so, too, was the absence of frustration, at least on this day.

The teachers prompted and coached without stop.

"Two in a bag."

"Good job, Jake."

"Robin, you are phenomenal!"

"Nice job!"

The language board said in its sci-fi voice, "I need a bag, please."

One boy had a hard time opening the Ziploc bag.

One girl was so slow it was as if she were floating underwater. Beside her a girl filled the bag without prompting or delay, then held up the bag, eyed it, placed it on the table, and very precisely, a fraction of an inch at a time, pressed down on the zip line until the bag was sealed. The whole process took a couple of minutes.

Meanwhile:

"One in each container!"

"You need to *ask* if you need more supplies."

"Dawn! Dawn!" This was my kid's familiar, maddening, attention-getting chime.

Dawn was busy with Jake, asking, "How many are in a bag? How *many,* Jake?" "Two."

"And how many are in *that* bag?"

Jake looked up, fastened his huge eyes on her.

"I'm running out of bags!" Rachel said. Then catching my eye, she gestured *come here* with her fingers.

I ignored her, and she went back to her task.

And then—here's the thing—everyone was at work. Except for the teachers' enthusiastic prompts, the room was quiet. There was no sign of discord or unhappiness, no sense that this was drudgery. These students were more focused than the kids in an average public-school class. They were working! They were engaged. And they kept at it for twenty minutes, until the first sorting job was done. The next step would be for them to put smaller tires in the same bags.

But first, break time. A chance to stretch or move about, get a drink of water, chat with their friends. One of the aides put on latex gloves, filled a huge syringe with milky-colored liquid, and squirted it into Robin's mouth. He gurgled and gagged: it was a messy, difficult process.

When Rachel found me, I asked what she was doing. "They have them putting in tires for other people," she said. "They have a lot of stuff for students to sort." Then she whipped out a bottle of purple nail polish from her pocket.

Her classmate, a dark-haired girl, dreamy and angelic-looking, approached, getting right up in my face to sign. I was embarrassed that I did not understand her, reminded that I was a foreigner in this country where my daughter spent most of her time.

At last she formed a word. "Mommy?" she asked.

"Yes, I'm Rachel's mom."

"Boots?" she asked.

I lifted up my pant cuff and showed her. "Yes," I said. "I'm wearing boots."

A boy came over to show me the mean-looking dog on the front of his T-shirt. "K-Mart!" he said. I'd already heard him tell the teacher where his mom got the shirt.

When break was over, the students were back in their seats for a second, shorter session. Dawn reminded them with the same short, crisply delivered sentences that they would be putting two little tires into a bag that already had two bigger tires. And then they were back to work.

When I told Dawn that I was impressed, she agreed that the kids had been working well. "We can't keep them supplied. Their rate and speed have really improved."

I *was* impressed.

I was also stunned—by all the effort it took to put two tires into a plastic bag, by the sight of my daughter with her peers, by the range of ability and disability in that room, the sheer diversity of this population we so blithely lumped together as having "special needs." But mostly what stayed with me was the diligent way the kids worked.

RACHEL AT WORK

On the way to see Michael Stoehr, who heads the career-education program, I thought how I felt when work goes well, when I have been so absorbed by my tasks, so "in the flow," that time vanishes. I thought about my sense of well-being at the end of a day like that, and how much I wanted that for Rachel, not because work per se would be good for her soul, not because I was pretending her life would resemble mine, but because when she was focused — playing Free Cell or solitaire on the computer, for instance — she was at peace. When we play Uno, one of the few games that fully engages her, she is fun to be with, her constant talking silenced at last.

So I was full of dreamy good cheer when I knocked on Michael Stoehr's door.

We talked about Dawn's class and some of the other work experiences Rachel has had at school — counting, sorting, housekeeping tasks. "One of her biggest difficulties is concentrating — just staying on task," he said. "She's distracted by what's going on around her." Though she was being considered for supported employment, it wasn't a sure thing.

In the world outside school — even in the world of supported employment — she would be expected to be "somewhat independent," he said. The job-coaching she would need was "pretty intense, pretty long-range. And at this point, the supports just aren't out there."

Supported employment wasn't a sure thing.

Sometimes reality hits like an ax.

3. Sometimes she talks too much; it's hard for either of us to know what she wants.

What did Rachel want? Maybe it was ridiculous the way we were pushing her to do so many things that were so difficult for her, I thought when I left Stoehr's office. Maybe she just didn't want to work. But if she didn't have a job, what would she do all day long when she was no longer in school?

In this era of self-determination and person-centered planning, I was supposed to be asking these kinds of questions. All the literature I got explaining the transition process urged me to view my child as a "total person," and make sure her desires were "at the heart of decision making." The materials prepared by the Allegheny County Department of Human Services, Office of Mental Retardation/Developmental Disabilities reminded me that self-determination is "a fundamental human right." People with mental retardation should have "the freedom to choose the services and supports they want, the authority to control limited resources and the responsibility for the decisions they make."

How can I respect Rachel's fundamental human right to choose what she will do after she is out of school without abandoning her to a world she cannot fully understand?

Well, there's conjecture: what I think she wants, based on my observations. And there are the dozens of questions about her likes and dislikes that I attempt to answer for her as honestly as I can when I fill out paperwork. And, I can't deny, there's my own will at work, since left to her own, Rachel would rather sit in front of a trough of potato chips and eat until she falls asleep than go to Special Olympics basketball. But I say, "She likes basketball" because when I spy on her from the doorway, I can see she's enjoying herself. I know I'm cheating, that *I* want her to play basketball and swim because it's good for her. Still, because I really do want to respect her desires, I sometimes set up my little microcassette tape recorder and interview her. I mentioned this to a friend once, and she was somewhat taken aback. "Why don't you just *talk* to her?" she asked.

I interview Rachel so I can hear her. In everyday life, she is so demanding, her nonstop talk so full of what I think of as sheer nothingness—endless questions about each move I make, about future plans, mostly to do with food, which I've answered dozens of times. Yes, I'll make dinner as soon as you hang up your jacket and use the bathroom. Yes (hang up your jacket). Yes (bathroom first). Yes (did you flush?) yes (did you wash your hands?) yes (with soap?) yes (you didn't flush!) yes. Her conversation is full of things that are real, overheard things that happened to someone else, things that are wrenchingly true.

If Rachel's incessant talking is both her prime means of communication and her strength—she can be funny and charming, full of personality—it is also her most profound, most unmanageable behavioral issue. She is, as one document states, "attention seeking, with a tendency to interrupt and begin talking about a non-related topic. . . . She is difficult to redirect."

Sometimes it is so noisy when I'm with her that I must expend a great amount of energy willing myself not to shriek at her to just shut up.

Sometimes I'm an earthmover, and she is the mountain. I am up there in my little cab, yelling, "Get a move on!" and ramming her.

When I interview her, I wait until she's out of the house before I replay the tape. Sometimes what I hear is how extraordinarily hard it is for her to process more than one or two simple, concrete questions before a tweeting bird or footsteps in another room set her off on a tangent. Sometimes I can sort out someone else's interests from her own. And sometimes in the silence of my room, apart from her, what I hear with great clarity is her heart's desire. Then I am close to all that makes her human. Listening to the tapes, I think about her in bed, lost beneath a huge gorilla and teddy bear and a dozen smaller stuffed animals. I think about her own, very clearly defined sense of "cool"—the hooded sweatshirt and sweatpants her sister chose for her birthday, which she sneaks out of the closet and tries to wear every day, even in summer. I think about the books she cannot read but insists upon getting at the library every Saturday and carrying everywhere, about her purple Mardi Gras beads. I think about her telling a friend that she wants to drink beer when she turns twenty-one.

I recall the day we were preparing for her first-ever sleepover guest and that, when I asked what she wanted to do with Jennie, she said, "Thnuggle." I think about the childish lisp that, given all the crucial therapies, all the urgent tasks she must master, we've never tried to correct, and this most human desire to be close to others, a desire that her incessant talking and her resistance to hygiene threaten to prevent.

I listen to the tapes and hear myself asking and asking what she wants, and I hear her say:

"I want to go on the bus."

"I want to be able to go out with a friend once in a while and do stuff."

"I want to see if I can get a cell phone, Ma."

"I want to look for an apartment."

I ask if she wants to have a job.

"Yes," she says. "Somewhere in this area."

What would she like to do?

"Look for something me and Jennie can do together."

I cue Rachel, try to get her to name some favorite jobs.

"Making dinner," she says. "Computer." "I like to look at the newspaper once in a while."

I back up to try to get her back on track. "What's my job?" I ask.

"Teaching," she says. "Writing."

"What about the JCC?" I ask. "What's your job there?"

"Working at the café."

What does she do there?

"Sell stuff to drink and eat. They have all different ice creams and all that stuff."

"What happens if a person comes and wants something?"

"They don't have any more sandwiches."

"So what happens if—"

"Listen! Listen. Just listen! They don't have any more sandwiches because they sold them all last time, and that's why we're doing this, because we don't have any more. We only have what's on the board."

Again I back up and try to redirect her. What does she do when the customers are gone?

"We clean up. The whole purpose is to clean up after we're doing selling candy and selling drinks and locking up machines. And we're doing that because we always have power-walking, but not today. With whatever her name is. She didn't show up, so Jennie left, and then I left."

I remind her that the confusion with power-walking was something that happened a few days ago. Maybe she can tell me about cleaning up.

"There's a big problem with the machines, usually."

What machines?

"The yellow-and-gray machines. The Popsicle machines, Ma. The ice-cream machines. They got locked up wrong yesterday by someone, and what happened was, after the fact that they had them locked up wrong was like a weird compliment, accomplishment, with like after this was going on it was fine, and then after that was—what are you writing down?"

Later I ask if she likes her job at the JCC.

"People talk to me too much, and I just can't stand it. It's hard for me to concentrate. It's better for me to do the dry cleaning, Mom. Better than the café."

Part of that statement is profoundly true. My daughter, with her relentless talking, is so terribly distractible that she cannot concentrate anywhere there is noise or conversation. But the dry cleaning, which she could nicely define ("It's where you take your clothes to the Laundromat, and you have to pay for it"), is something she knows only because her friend had some with him one day. Dry cleaning is like drinking beer at twenty-one and going to college—things that others have or discuss, rather than a wish from her own heart.

A few days after my visit to Rachel's work-production class, I asked her what jobs she was doing in school.

"I'm not doing the cups anymore," she said.

"What do you do in the mornings?"

"Only the paper towels."

And what did she do with the paper towels?

"Put them in the holder. In the paper-towel bin."

"And what else do you do?"

"Plates. We fill plates. Although here's the big part, Ma—are you ready for it?—we're selling chips and stuff like that now."

And so we had moved in time and place, from school, perhaps on that day, to her job at Café J on a nameless day in a month that fell as randomly as a snowflake.

4. There is no safety net.

Though Barbara Milch's official title is division director of children, family and youth, I think of her as the person who has helped make the JCC of Greater Pittsburgh into a near-perfect world, where people with special needs are a visible part of the community. She spearheaded the current programs that make it possible for kids with special needs to be included in after-school programs and summer camps. Nor have teens and adults been forgotten: Most of what Rachel does outside of school—her chance to go to a play, see a ball game, be with friends—originates here at the JCC because of Barbara's efforts.

The café was initially a joint project Barbara initiated with Jewish Residential Services to employ people with chronic mental illness as a primary diagnosis. When funding from a startup grant ran out, she was able to put anyone in the job. Thus Rachel and her cohort (and their therapeutic staff-support people) were given shifts.

In my some-job-somewhere phase, I took great pleasure in seeing Rachel in her red apron, wearing her staff badge. The JCC is a busy community center with nearly fifteen thousand members. Lots of people I know who use the athletic facilities or have kids in child care stop at the café and are served by Rachel. It made me feel good to think of my daughter out in the world this way, not merely some mysterious, hidden-away, half-grown child I was rumored to have.

Now that I am looking beyond the gloss made up of relief, gratitude and fatigue, I am forced to ask: What will happen when Rachel has no TSS?

This is not doomsday thinking. I've already contested the proposed termination of funding for this costly behavior-management therapy, and though I was successful, still I know that these services are designed to "fade," even though her issues may never be completely resolved. Rachel cannot work in the café without this assistance—not for the foreseeable future, at least.

She's learned a lot since she began at the café. She knows the prices of everything and that the customers should check the board to see what is being offered that day. She has memorized the sequence of tasks necessary to close down the café.

Skills are not enough. Before this spring I imagined Rachel's future based merely on her strengths (she's gregarious) and deficits (poor vision, poor fine-motor skills). But I had failed to regard the rest of her. It was as if her behavior and attention issues were things that made it hard for *me* to live with her but that would not impact her ability to work. I had somehow failed to integrate what I had known all along: The greatest obstacle to her working is her distractibility.

At Café J she has "difficulty balancing appropriate socialization with her peers with the need to focus and concentrate on the demands of working in the café," I read. "She continues to ask for assistance with skills she has mastered and can successfully manipulate various JC staff to engage in 'over-helping.' Often she does not want to follow through with requests to complete her responsibilities for the café."

And didn't she herself manage to tell me exactly why she was struggling? *People talk to me too much, and I just can't stand it. It's hard for me to concentrate.*

Barbara has tried to reassure me. "She will always have a home at the JCC."

But at this time, in the spring of 2002, I am forced to wonder—*a home doing what?*

Though I cannot underestimate the importance of community, neither can I bear to imagine Rachel wandering the corridors of the JCC, trying to engage unwitting strangers in meaningless talk—unwitting strangers because, if she stays long enough, only strangers will not know to avoid her.

Wandering, following people, trying to engage them—this is what Rachel's day will look like if she cannot be trained for supported employment. It is what she's like at home, that most unstructured place, where everyone else is off doing something—reading, paying bills, talking on the phone, walking up and down the stairs. When we are home for too long together, Rachel's calls for attention, her birdlike *Ma? Mommy? Ma?* is so insistent I choose the most distant part of the house just to escape her.

Michael Stoehr warned me that the supports Rachel gets at school are entitlements mandated by law, that after school these supports are often unavailable. At present they aren't there for millions of individuals in the United States with mild mental retardation. Only 7–23 percent of these people are employed full-time, in part because of the inadequacy of vocational training. Rachel, with her greater needs, is in far greater jeopardy. At school and at the JCC, she has staff at her side nearly all the time. In the outside world, it's different.

"Some agencies will say they're going to follow her, but the reality is they'll provide support for about a month or two," Stoehr says. "After that they're looking for results and turnaround, ready to pull out. . . . It's a very unfair system. There are not a lot of easy answers or nice solutions."

I know this is true, just as I understand that distractibility is Rachel's most serious handicap. And yet I have seen her quiet down. I have watched her sit at the computer for long stretches of time. And it makes me wonder. In this era adaptations are made so people can learn and travel and work. There are language boards and gigs and orthotics, bicycles that can be pedaled by hand, computers that speak, lifts to bring wheelchairs onto buses. Must I believe that an adaptation can never be made for Rachel? Must I say that she will never be able to work? If I do that, I am left imagining my daughter wandering aimlessly, trying to engage people, unwittingly pushing them away—a lonely, marginalized person.

5. Take a nap and then wake up.

So you're tired. So what, I need to remind myself. Take a nap, and while you're sleeping, dream some sweet dreams. And then wake up.

You know what she needs. Now search for it. If you can't find it, you'll have to make it happen.

It's exhausting, but what can I say?

She has her work, and I have mine.

•

Jane Bernstein is an associate professor of English and creative writing at Carnegie-Mellon University. She is the author of three books, and her numerous essays have appeared in the New York Times Magazine, Glamour, Self, Poets & Writers, *and other publications.*

Breast Cancer #2

Margaret Overton

∽

I t's 5 o'clock, and the long cases are over. There's just one more to go—the last of the day. One of my partners throws open the operating-room door and stands facing me with his mask down around his neck, his surgeon's gown backward and hanging open over dirty scrubs, his pants pulled low by double pagers at his waist.

"Want me to do your last case?" he asks.

I consider saying yes—my shoulders ache. I'm getting a cold, and I've been here since 6:30 A.M. "Nah, but thanks." I know the case will be short. Better to save up favors for when the kids are sick or have a basketball game.

Anyway it's a simple case. Pretty straightforward. Not even a general anesthetic but intravenous sedation for a central line insertion, probably for chemo or something. Young patient—a young woman—a surgeon I like, nurses I enjoy working with. Easy as can be, no more than an hour. I draw up drugs into fresh syringes. The surgeon will inject local anesthetic into her skin. I pick up the phone in the OR, call home and tell my older daughter I won't be too late tonight. She says she needs help with math homework.

In presurgery, where the patients wait with family members, I flip open my patient's chart to the nursing admission form. The patient's name is Onica M.; the diagnosis is breast cancer, recurrent. The hospital stamps her identification card on the right-hand corner of each page of her chart. The stamp shows her age as 039. This distinguishes her from patients named Onica M. with recurrent breast cancer who are, perhaps, 139? I, too, am 039.

Onica lies on a metal cart, dressed in the universal uniform of the patient—the hospital gown that snaps at the shoulders and ties in the back. She's covered by the usual institutional white sheet, over which the institutional white blanket has been placed to prevent the institutional chill. She's been stripped of her clothes, jewelry, nail polish and makeup; her distinguishing characteristics are now elemental—she's allowed to maintain her general build, hair color, facial features. Soon we'll cover her head with a disposable hat, and she'll look almost like us—except of course for the ways in which terminal disease has transformed her. That's always the giveaway.

When I reach out to shake her hand, I notice she's tiny, thin, petite—a sprite of a person. Big-boned and tall, more like my father than my mother, I've always envied petite women, the way they constantly surprise you by being more than they seem. During adolescence I stared at my thighs and longed to be shorter, as short as most other girls, short enough to be normal. Now I no longer mind the height, but I still take note of what I'll never be.

Onica's skin is light tan and her hair light brown. She reaches out to grasp my hand with her small, bony one, holds it fiercely in hers, grips mine a moment longer than necessary. Her hand makes me think of a crunchy Middle Eastern delicacy: the fig birds they deep-fry and eat whole. When she releases me, her arm remains outstretched, suspended, floating in space, as if she isn't sure she should have let go. We smile at each other, or rather, I do; she doesn't smile so much as grin. Onica is cute, a pixie, a pert, perky woman who might have been a member of the pompon squad in high school, like Annette Sullivan or Sherry Kopinsky. Someone everyone liked. Dimples crease her cheeks when she grins. I shake hands with her father, who sits quietly beside her, staring at nothing, looking prosperous but lost, ineffably sad.

He kisses Onica's cheek, then we leave him in presurgery and wheel Onica back to the operating room, where I attach the monitors—ECG electrodes, blood-pressure cuff, pulse oximeter. I start giving her drugs. Lidocaine, then fentanyl, then midazolam. I plug in the propofol infusion, set the pump to her body weight and a low dose. I can judge the effects of the medication more easily if she's talking, so while the drugs are starting to work, I ask her questions. I pay attention to the pace and cadence of her answers, wait for the speech to gradually slur. Everyone's tolerance is different, so I titrate the drugs to the desired effect.

"Are you married?" I ask, holding her arm above the IV site, rubbing gently to take the sting out of the medicine.

"Oh, yeah," she answers, her voice bright with enthusiasm, "and I've got two kids, a boy and a girl."

"How old are they?"

"My son is eleven, and my daughter's nine."

"So they're what—in third and fifth?"

"Third and sixth," she answers, her words slightly thick, coming a little bit slower. "They're two and a half years apart, but three years in school." I look down and smile behind my facemask. Once again I see that grin—a quick twitch of tense facial muscles. Onica uses her dimples wisely, I think. She uses them to hide her fear, perhaps, or anger or sadness. In truth I don't know what she hides. I can't even imagine, so I slide another milligram of midazolam into her IV.

"What sports do they play?"

"Douglas, my son, well, Douglas . . . likes . . . soccer . . ."

Her eyes drift shut, and I nod to Maylie, the circulating nurse. She can begin the prep.

Maylie brings the prep stand close to the OR table. She folds the cotton blanket down to Onica's waist, refastens the safety belt on top of it. She removes the hospital gown, unsnapping it at the shoulders and turning it down to the waist. Despite the noise of the monitors, I hear Maylie's gasp. On Onica's chest, in place of breasts, which I knew she didn't have, sit two raw, lumpy, ulcerative masses. Scarred, puckered, with purple draining from angry red, these things disfigure her small body and silently scream *cancer.* I turn away, pull down my mask, and take a deep breath. Mercifully, amazingly, there is no odor. After a moment I look back and meet Maylie's tired eyes. Our gazes are drawn back against our wills to Onica.

"What . . . ?" Our scrub nurse, Paula, stops speaking, looks at me.

I shake my head. Though her eyes are closed, our patient is technically awake.

Gish, the general surgeon, enters the OR with hands raised and dripping. Paula hands him a towel, and as he dries his hands, he walks toward me and leans close.

"She had a TRAM flap breast reconstruction elsewhere," he whispers, "then a recurrence of her cancer. She got irradiated, and the flap broke down. That's all scar tissue and cancer." He backs away and looks straight at me. "Nice, huh?"

I sit down at the head of the OR table, touch Onica on the shoulder. "How you doing?" I ask. "You okay?"

She murmurs an assent, and once again, a slight grin appears and disappears. Her eyes remain shut. I stand up to affix the drapes, give Onica an additional bolus of propofol before Gish injects the local anesthetic into her skin. I whisper, "You'll feel a little sting now, as the numbing medicine goes in."

She barely flinches with the needle stick. I sit back down to continue my charting, observing Onica frequently to make sure she stays sleepy and unaware throughout the procedure. I listen to the rhythmic pattern of the monitors, the buzz of the electrocautery unit, while another part of me hurtles through space, through time, forward blindly, without any understanding of how movement occurs, entangled in the flawed harness of the helping profession. Though there are many layers to this job, the horror is a small part, a part that can be ignored, if you know how, that is, if you're good at it. I am a professional trained to function within an official, circumscribed vocabulary. The words I need—right now—to describe this exact moment don't exist within that lexicon.

Here's the thing. I absorb horror only in snippets, in quotas, one at a time, day after day. I preserve their essences, tell myself I will attend to them later, after the homework—perhaps I even mean it—but then another patient comes along. There's another job to do, another mess to slog through, and fatigue sets in; life sets in, and I don't do it. Not right, anyway. Not well enough. Part of this is self-protection. The other part, I've come to understand, is that compassion ultimately fails. How else can it be? I take care of patients when I am tired and alert and proud of my children and angry with my husband and upset because the radiator pipe broke and flooded my kitchen and when I am worried about the dog's rash. I have, after all, a job to do. I cannot permit immobilization. But on certain days with certain patients—she is 039, like me—I cannot help but see the whole of it.

I look back down at Onica, at the half-grin she wears even in repose. I remember the first TRAM flap I saw, and the anger comes rushing back to me. I've hated that plastic surgeon ever since. Does anger assuage survivor guilt? Perhaps my feelings are political, leftovers from a feminist upbringing. Who but a man would be clever enough to imagine transforming womanhood in the first place—relocating abdominal muscles upward to re-create breast tissue while performing a concomitant tummy tuck? Massive surgery, long hours of blood loss and anesthesia, undoubtedly sold on the premise that one surgery fixes you right up—good as new, better even. Then the cancer recurs—of course it does—in our patient, this young mother of two who will not see her children grow up but will watch them as they watch her suffer and die a slow death with little or no dignity.

In the recovery room, Onica is awake again and cheerful. I stand at her bedside and say nothing, just fiddle with the wires connecting her to the monitors. I ask mundane questions: what her husband does, where she grew up. I do not ask the questions I want to ask: Do you have a family history? What asshole plastic surgeon talked you into this abomination? How do you discuss the cancer with your kids? I do not ask, though I know she would tell me. It would be so easy to plunder her medical history. Onica M., with the grin for others, would tell me all her secrets, answer the questions I have no right to ask. But I don't ask. Someday perhaps I'll learn a language in which compassion does not fail or intrude or strip a sick woman of her strength or self-protection, a language in which compassion thrives, despite this gilded vocabulary. Maybe someday I will learn that language; I do not know it now.

My pager goes off yet again. Both daughters now need help with their math homework. Still I sit beside Onica until she leaves the recovery room to go back to her father, her family, her life and the end of her thirty-ninth year.

•

Margaret Overton is a physician practicing anesthesia in the Chicago area. She recently completed her MFA in writing at the School of the Art Institute of Chicago and is at work on a memoir.

The Burden of Baby Boy Smith

Helena Studer

◌

On a warm, sunny morning in July, I watched a baby die. I stood in Operating Room 2 of the obstetrics floor with my hands clenched at my sides, fighting every instinct I had, not to save a full-term baby boy.

As a doctor, I was trained to save lives. But to employ heroic measures to try to save this baby's life only meant prolonging his death. This baby was born with Potter syndrome, a rare genetic abnormality incompatible with life. *Smith's Recognizable Patterns of Human Malformations*, a genetics textbook, coldly and clinically denotes the disease as dysmorphic facies, pulmonary hypoplasia, renal agenesis. Simply, in plain language, this baby had a misshapen face and no working lungs or kidneys.

Two hours before this moment, I had been asked by the obstetrician to attend a high-risk delivery in the OR. He told me the mother was being induced because the baby was full-term, which normally would not mean a high-risk delivery—except the obstetrician already knew this baby had Potter syndrome. I was surprised that the mother had chosen to go full-term with this baby, knowing his diagnosis. But it became clear she was holding on to hope when she asked me repeatedly before delivery, "Doctor, will you do everything possible if he looks normal?" I assured her I would do everything appropriate no matter what happened. It was a tough promise to keep.

As I looked at the baby's tiny, malformed face, I reminded myself of the Hippocratic Oath: "First, do no harm." Although these exact words do not appear in the original Oath, which is still recited in unison by medical school graduates around the country during commencement every May, that's the Oath's overriding and most compelling message. "First, do no harm" repeated over and over in my head but gave me no comfort.

I wrapped the baby carefully in a pink-and-blue-striped baby blanket and cradled him as I walked over to his parents. I placed him in his mother's arms and left his parents with their grief. They held him until his heart stopped beating. At 11:15 A.M. of the same sunny day, I put my stethoscope to his chest and pronounced him dead. I did no harm. But I felt profound helplessness and sorrow.

Three months later, I questioned myself even more. To tell the rest of my story, I have changed the names and minor characteristics of everyone involved (patients, families, colleagues) to protect their identities.

Laurie ran into the nursing station shouting my name.

"Dr. Studer! You have to come to the OR right now! Dr. Sullivan needs you stat! There's a baby in trouble!"

I was out of my chair and running out of the pediatric ward before she finished. Laurie, the nurse manager of both the pediatric and OB/GYN units, rarely panicked and never ran. The sight was disconcerting. Her short, dark hair, normally perfectly coiffed, was in disarray, her round, pleasant face creased in consternation. We both rushed down the corridor towards the delivery rooms.

"What happened?!"

"Dr. Sullivan's doing a stat C-section! He can't find the baby's heart rate! He thinks it's a uterine rupture!"

"Oh my God! How long has the baby been down?"

"We don't know—about five minutes at this point. Dr. Sullivan is scrubbing right now. He wants you to be ready when he gets the baby out."

Uterine rupture is a death sentence for a baby. When a pregnant woman's uterus ruptures, blood no longer flows to the baby. The umbilical cord, the lifeline which carries in oxygen and nutrients and carries out waste, no longer functions. A baby's brain cannot be deprived of oxygen for very long before there is irreparable damage. No one really knows how long that takes, but five minutes was already too long.

I left Laurie to run into the women's locker room. I changed out of my street clothes into scrubs; earrings flew onto the floor as I yanked my shirt over my head. All the while thinking: *I'm not a neonatologist, I'm a general pediatrician! What am I doing here?* But as a pediatric hospitalist employed by a well-known Children's Hospital, I was required to attend deliveries at this affiliate hospital when requested by the obstetricians. The closest neonatologist was an hour away.

I peered through the window of Operating Room 2. Dennis Sullivan, the obstetrician, was already cutting. I put a mask on my face and walked into the OR.

"Who is that? Is that you, Helena?" Dennis's voice echoed off the cold tile walls.

"Yes, Dennis, it's me." I was unrecognizable behind my mask; hairnet, shoe covers, and scrubs hid the rest of me.

I carefully kept to the periphery of the operating table to avoid contaminating anything. Preserving the integrity of the sterile field, specifically the area where the surgeon operates, is a priority. Prevention of infection, one of the worst complications from surgery, starts in the OR.

"Thanks for coming so quickly. I would have given you more notice if I could, but this happened rather suddenly," Dennis apologized as he turned for a quick nod at me.

"She was a VBAC at full-term that was doing great, then suddenly she started hemorrhaging. We lost the fetal heart rate. The baby will be down fifteen or twenty minutes before we can get him out." His speech was pressured as he operated swiftly.

෴

I blanched at the time frame. Twenty minutes—a lifetime for a baby.

I walked to the neonatal resuscitation area in the far corner of the OR. Donna, a delivery room nurse, had already turned on the warmer above the neonatal resuscitation tray. We called it a "tray" because, although technically a bed, it was the size of a large tray with a thin, plastic-covered foam mattress surrounded on three sides by shallow glass walls to stop a baby from rolling off. Ordinarily it was used just to warm the baby as he adjusted to life outside the womb. Most babies need only to be dried and stimulated as they make the transition to the external world. This baby would need much more.

The digital controls on the column supporting the tray and the warmer in the overhang blinked furiously.

"What size ET tube would you like ready?" Donna asked.

"Oh, probably a 3.5 since he's full-term but have a 3.0 ready in case he turns out to be smaller. May I have the straight blade also, just in case?" I asked as I took inventory of things I would need to resuscitate this baby. Donna placed the two different sizes of endotracheal (ET) tubes and the straight-blade laryngoscope I requested next to a pile of warmed baby blankets, a suction catheter, a curved-blade laryngoscope, and a bag-mask ventilator with an infant face mask already on the tray.

Some physicians prefer the straight "blade," or flat, narrow metal tongue of a laryngoscope, over the curved blade, claiming the straight blade gives a better view of the vocal cords. Therefore it is easier to slip the ET, or breathing tube, between the vocal cords and into the trachea: the pathway of oxygen into the lungs. I didn't subscribe to this theory; I wanted all my options. I opened up the blankets and layered several on the tray so that as each blanket became wet and dirty, we could remove just the top one and a clean one would already be in place. We could not afford to waste time.

"Have you called Respiratory?" I was referring to the respiratory therapist who could assist us in airway management.

"It's Margie today. She has an emergency in the Cardiac ICU, but she'll be here as soon as she can," Donna replied, and then asked hesitantly, "Should I take anything out of the code cart?"

"You should probably get one dose each of epi and bicarb ready. I hate to waste the doses, but we don't have time to futz if we need them," I answered as calmly as I could.

Epinephrine is needed to jump-start the heart if it is not beating, and sodium bicarbonate increases body pH to combat the acidosis that results from lack of oxygen and blood flow. I kept repeating the mantra "ABC, ABC, ABC" in my head. Airway, Breathing, Circulation are the core principles of Basic Life Support skills taught to interns in the first week of their training to prepare them for the emergencies they will surely encounter in the course of their careers. This was an emergency. Vaginal Birth after Caesarean, or VBAC, was a fairly common occurrence these days. Many women felt they missed out on part of the experience of giving birth if they had a C-section. Encouraged by their obstetricians, though not without risks, women were trying VBACs. Unfortunately, for this mother, the less than 1 percent risk of uterine rupture had come true. Her baby was in danger.

Compulsively, I checked and rechecked my equipment. Several times, I squeezed the blue bag of the bag-mask ventilator with the tiny face mask pressed against my palm. I was trying to make sure the pressure generated was adequate but not so much that it would blow out the baby's lungs. I clicked the laryngoscope open to form a metal "L" to see if the built-in light was working. Without a light, I could not guide the ET tube past the vocal cords and into the trachea. I pressed the thin plastic tip of the suction catheter against my finger, feeling the gentle pull of suction. Mucus or meconium could obstruct my view of his airway and would need to be removed. I stretched the back of my hand up towards the radiant heat source of the warmer, even though I could feel the heat down on the tray. Keeping the baby warm would be crucial in maintaining his desired core temperature of 98.6 degrees Fahrenheit. I scrutinized the size of the ET tubes against the packaging and recounted the blankets, worried we did not have enough.

"Why don't you scrub now, we're getting close," Dennis advised.

Fighting my panic and the urge to run out of the OR, I walked to the scrub sink right outside the door. Meticulously, I scoured my fingers, hands and arms with antibacterial soap and a brush; the smell of betadine was so pungent, I turned my head away. I reentered the OR with my arms flexed and my hands held away from my body, water dripping onto the floor. Despite the urgency of this situation, rituals still had to be obeyed. Going through the routine, methodical process of disinfection helped to keep my anxiety under control. One of the OR nurses passed me a sterile towel to dry my hands. I carefully put on the sterile gown, and she helped me tie it; she held the sterile gloves open as I shoved my fingers into them. Finally, she handed me the sterile baby blanket in which I would carry the baby to the tray. I waited quietly, staring at the clock.

After what seemed like a really long time, Dennis asked, "Are you ready? The baby is coming out."

I stepped closer to the operating table and held out the blanket. Dennis dropped a limp baby into my arms. The baby was a perfectly formed little boy except for his color: blue so dark it was navy. I never saw such a shade. I knew he was dead. I ran over and plopped him on the resuscitation tray. Placing the face mask of the bag-mask ventilator over his mouth and nose, I quickly squeezed the bag, attempting to force oxygen into his lungs.

"Start chest compressions, please," I instructed Donna in a rush.

She placed two fingers on the baby's sternum and rapidly pushed down.

Suzanne, my favorite nurse in the newborn nursery, suddenly appeared at my elbow. "What do you need me to do?"

I nodded gratefully, "Can you hand me the suction and have the laryngoscope ready? I'm going to intubate."

Suzanne quickly gave me the suction catheter as I put down the bag-mask ventilator. I pushed the catheter into the baby's mouth and sucked out mucus, then quickly took the laryngoscope, clicked it open and thrust it into the baby's mouth and pulled up, lifting the soft palate and looking for the epiglottis. It popped into view. The vocal cords followed.

"A 3.5 please." I held out my hand, my eyes fixed on the vocal cords.

Suzanne slapped the ET tube into my right hand and I rapidly inserted it between the vocal cords. Stabilizing the heel of my left hand on the baby's forehead, I gripped the ET tube between my thumb and forefinger, keeping it from slipping too far down his trachea and ventilating only one lung instead of both. Before I could ask, Suzanne tore the face mask off the bag-mask ventilator, clamped the ventilator on top of the ET tube, and pressed the blue bag quickly. The baby's chest rose symmetrically, indicating that oxygen was getting into both lungs. Suzanne continued ventilating as I taped the ET tube into place. The baby's face was no longer blue; a tinge of pink crept up his neck.

"Do we have a heart rate?" I needed to know.

Donna checked his umbilical stump for a pulse. She shook her head. "No."

She resumed chest compressions and I took over rhythmically squeezing the ventilator bag.

"How long has it been?" My eyes were glued on the clock, wanting to know the length of resuscitation.

"Ninety seconds so far."

It seemed an eternity.

"Let's give a dose of epi, please." My trepidation was growing with each squeeze of the blue bag.

The mantra in my head continued: ABC, ABC, ABC. Airway, Breathing, Circulation.

We had established an airway, and now he was breathing with our help. Circulation was next; his heart needed to pump blood. Unlike adults, most babies during resuscitation respond very quickly to oxygenation and ventilation. Once oxygen is delivered to the lungs, it triggers the heart to start beating. I concentrated on the rise of the baby's chest, willing his heart to beat with every squeeze of the blue bag. No response.

I heard the chaos around me, but the shouting sounded like it was in the distance instead of next to my ear. What echoed in my head was: *What am I doing?* Doubt about the implications of my actions clamored to be heard, but I refused to listen. I crowded everything out except the baby in front of me. I saw Margie run into the delivery room dragging a ventilator machine behind her; out of the corner of my eye I saw the syringe with epi fall out of Donna's hand as if in slow motion. I saw Suzanne turn to the code cart, its bright red color blurring into the background as she reached for a vial of epi and drew it up in a syringe—less than fifteen seconds. I popped the ventilator bag off and Suzanne shot the epi down the ET tube. We continued ventilating with chest compressions for what seemed an excruciatingly long time. I was considering a second round of epinephrine, as well as bicarbonate this time, when Donna shouted in excitement.

"I have a heart rate!"

"What is it?" Disbelief in my voice.

Suzanne squeezed his umbilical stump. "It's less than 60 but it's coming up!"

Relief swept over me. I closed my eyes. *Thank God.* I heard clapping and congratulations. I put my stethoscope on his chest. His heart was beating and struggling to go higher. Soon it was beating at over 100 times per minute, more like a normal baby's.

"Okay, let's get him into the nursery. We'll continue from there," I directed as Margie hooked up his ET tube to the ventilator machine. I glanced at the clock: less than five minutes of resuscitation. I let a ray of hope into the darkness of my thoughts. Maybe he was going to be okay.

We wheeled the baby, with machinery in tow, down the short hallway to the newborn nursery. As I entered, the wailing of newborns hit me like a wall, asserting their life force and demanding attention.

This baby lay motionless as we pushed him into a single, glass-walled room in the middle of the nursery. The room's occupant and monitoring equipment could be seen from the far corners of the nursery; it was occasionally used as a makeshift neonatal intensive care unit (NICU).

Laurie rushed in. "I was watching from the window with the father, trying to tell him everything was okay. He's frightened. He and his wife are asking about the baby. What should I tell them?"

I shook my head, not knowing what to say. "We've given him epi, he's intubated on a ventilator. He's pretty sick and we have a lot of work to do. I guess you should tell his parents that he is sick, but stable. You should prepare them for the fact that he's going to be transported to Children's NICU as soon as possible."

The newborn nursery had neither the equipment nor the staff to be a neonatal intensive care unit. And I was not a neonatologist.

Suzanne peeked out from the glass room. "Margie says his blood gas is not so good."

She handed me a narrow slip of paper: pH- 6.8, pO2- 95, pCO2- 35. Normal body pH approximates 7.4. I had expected metabolic acidosis because of the lack of oxygen and blood flow, but a pH of 6.8 was incompatible with life. But then, he had been dead for at least twenty minutes.

"Okay, let's give him some bicarb and recheck his blood gas in half an hour." My voice flat, displaying no emotion. I had to move on to the next task.

I turned to Laurie, "Please tell his parents I'll come speak to them as soon as I can. But first, he needs line access. I have to put in UA and UV lines."

I was referring to umbilical arterial and umbilical venous lines. Babies are born with umbilical arteries and veins, blood vessels which in-utero provided a direct link to their hearts from their mothers. If babies are born with tenuous medical conditions, physicians can access these same vessels to give intravenous medications, electrolytes, water, sugar and to monitor directly the functioning of their hearts. The fact that this baby needed UA and UV lines was yet another indication of how sick he was. He could not breathe on his own, nor depend on his heart to keep pumping, much less feed himself.

As I threaded the catheter up the umbilical artery towards his heart, I became acutely aware of my distaste for this task. Piercing the arm, leg, abdomen or spine of babies with a needle had never bothered me before the birth of my daughter less than a year earlier. I justified that I needed to test their blood or urine or cerebrospinal fluid by any means possible. I told myself: I'm doing this for their own good. But now, I was squeamish about sticking needles into babies. I could not explain it; the need to obtain fluids for testing or to gain intravenous access was no less critical, but it suddenly seemed cruel. Especially to this baby.

After stripping off the sterile gown and gloves I used to place the UA and UV lines, I sat down at a counter in the section of the newborn nursery designated as the nursing station and stared at blank sheets of paper. Surrounded by persistent cries of newborns, I tried to ignore the voice in my head: *What have I done?* The adrenaline which had kept me going suddenly dissipated. I was exhausted. I wondered when David, another pediatric hospitalist, was coming to relieve me. I felt like I couldn't last until then.

But there was work to do. I picked up the phone to call Children's Hospital for help. I had a detailed conversation with the neonatologist, and she agreed to send helicopter transport instead of slower ambulance transport. I was writing in Baby Boy Smith's chart when I felt a hand on my shoulder. I looked up at Dennis Sullivan.

"How's the baby doing?" He sat down next to me, folding his towering, lanky body to fit the chair. He pushed his sparse, graying hair away from his forehead as he put his elbows down on the writing counter.

"Okay. His blood gas looks good for the most part, and he's on minimal ventilator settings. And we got in the lines we needed." I tried to sound optimistic.

"I talked to his parents. They would like to talk to you, too. I told them you were busy, but I would appreciate you taking some time with them when you can," Dennis said quietly.

"I will, Dennis. I just got off the phone with Children's—they're coming to get him. I wanted to write down the events of his resuscitation before the helicopter gets here, otherwise it's going to sound all confused." I defended my reluctance.

"I know," he nodded. "You have your hands full. I'll just write my note to complete his chart before copies are made for transport."

But he made no move to write anything. Instead he sat hunched over a blank piece of paper, staring into space.

"Dennis, are you okay?" I touched his arm.

He turned to face me, "Sorry—I'm not used to this. Normally, I'm the one congratulating the dad as he passes me a cigar. I'm just feeling sorry for myself. In twenty years of delivering babies, I've never had a uterine rupture. I keep thinking: If only I didn't let her go VBAC."

His face aged before me; the lines around his eyes deepened and the intensity of his gaze diminished to a faded blue.

"I'm sorry." My words hung in the air, inadequate against his anguish.

"Do you know what's going to happen to the baby?" he asked, his face earnest.

"Well, he's going to be in Children's NICU for a while, weaning off the vent, starting feeds . . ."

"No," he shook his head impatiently. "I mean, what's going to *happen* to him?"

I had been avoiding this moment. I did not want to define the consequences of birth asphyxia. I didn't even want to think about it.

Suzanne interrupted. "He's seizing. What do you want to give him?"

I looked at the clock hanging above the counter. Less than an hour since resuscitation and he was having seizures. Things were definitely going from bad to worse.

"Jesus." I stood up, weary. I felt defeated. "Let's give him a dose of Ativan. I have to call Children's back. I don't know what to load him with to stop the seizures—probably Phenobarb." Ativan, a sedative, is used as an anticonvulsant in acute situations, and Phenobarbital is the most common anticonvulsant given long-term in children.

I walked into the glass room and stared at his twitching form. His tiny body, with tubes sticking out everywhere and hooked up to machinery to keep him alive, lay in classic surrender pose. His head was turned to one side; his legs splayed open; his arms flexed at almost ninety-degree angles with his fingers curled. Defenseless.

"I better go talk to his parents," I sighed. I could not delay the conversation any longer.

෴

My pink rubber clogs made small squeaking noises against the tile floor of the maternity ward. I knocked on room 1311.

"Come in," a muffled woman's voice called out.

I took a deep breath and entered. In a hospital bed, a woman reclined on a mound of pillows. She struggled to sit up, her pale face swollen, her long hair matted and limp. Next to her stood a slight man dwarfed by his brown jacket, denim overalls, and baseball cap. All showed signs of wear and dirt. I assumed he was a farmer. The town surrounding the hospital was still very much a tight-knit community of surviving family farms, just beginning to experience the suburban sprawl of the "big city." People still knew each other by name, had had the same neighbors for decades. When I first started working at the hospital, one wisecracking Emergency Room physician joked I was more likely to see a child because of a tractor accident than an asthma attack.

"Hi, I'm Dr. Studer, one of the pediatricians here at the hospital."

The man extended his hand. "I'm Joe and this here is my wife, Mary."

The woman nodded weakly from her bed.

"Nice to meet you." I shook his hand. "I wish it were in better circumstances . . ." I did not get the chance to finish.

"How's my baby?" she interrupted.

I worded my answer carefully. "He's stable. He has a breathing tube; he is on a ventilator that breathes for him. And we've placed intravenous lines to give him medications and fluids. We're monitoring his lungs and other organs like his heart and kidneys by checking his blood work. So far, everything looks good."

"Is he going to be all right?" Her wide gray eyes locked with mine.

I evaded her question, "So far the blood work looks good. His lungs and heart are working and he's stable." I paused before continuing. "But I have to tell you just now in the nursery, he started having seizures."

They both looked at me blankly. I waited for this information to sink in.

"What does that mean?" the father asked, confusion on his face.

Again, I was careful with my answer. "Your baby's brain was deprived of oxygen for twenty minutes. We don't know precisely how that will affect his brain. But it is not unusual for seizures to occur when a brain is deprived of oxygen. We are treating him for seizures with medication and, of course, we'll watch him carefully."

I prayed they would not ask me what the long-term effects of oxygen deprivation were on a baby's brain. The data on birth asphyxia are pretty ominous.

Birth asphyxia results in brain damage that can range from mild mental retardation to coma with life support. The most common manifestations of brain damage are mental retardation, cerebral palsy, hearing loss, and visual impairment. The U.S. Centers for Disease Control reported in January 2004 that "estimated lifetime costs in 2003 dollars are expected to total $51.2 billion for persons born in 2000 with mental retardation, $11.5 billion for persons with cerebral palsy." Furthermore, "average lifetime costs per person were estimated at $1,014,000 for persons with mental retardation, $921,000 for persons with cerebral palsy, $417,000 for persons with hearing loss, and $566,000 for persons with vision impairment." Of course, the study, intended to quantify the economic cost to the country of these "developmental disabilities," did not account for the human or emotional cost to the patient, family members, or the hospital staff that care for these patients. I knew too many children with devastating consequences of birth asphyxia to dismiss this particular cost.

I thought about Joshua Bennet, a nine-year-old who had recently died. Joshua suffered birth asphyxia. His mother told me that his umbilical cord had twisted around his neck, cutting off all oxygen to his brain for over ten minutes. As a result, Joshua had brain damage in the form of seizures, mental retardation, cerebral palsy, hearing loss and visual impairment. His mother tried to keep Joshua at home. She said she even quit her job to accommodate Joshua's needs. But finally she broke down; by the time Joshua turned six, she could no longer handle his mounting nursing care and medication needs. Every weekend she visited him at a long-term-care facility for children with disabilities.

I got to know Joshua and his mother because he was frequently transferred to the pediatric floor of the hospital because of intractable seizures and aspiration pneumonia. On his third admission for pneumonia with deteriorating lung function and increasing seizures, I brought up "Do Not Resuscitate" (DNR) orders with his mother. She sat by Joshua's bedside holding his hand. He lay still in a blue hospital gown, his eyes closed, unresponsive to her touch. Minutes ago his body had been contorted by a seizure which alternately stiffened and jerked his limbs, arching his back. Now he moaned, his fine blond hair damp with sweat, his cheeks flushed, thin blue veins prominent on his white closed eyelids, his thin body covered with a white hospital sheet. His mother told me she prayed that God would end his suffering. Unable to stop the tears coursing down her face, she signed the form which allowed her son to die. Five months later, she buried him in their family plot.

Anita Rogers was another "frequent flyer." Pediatric residents at Children's Hospital gave that name to neurologically devastated children who were hospitalized frequently because of their fragile medical conditions. It reflected accurately just how often Anita was in the hospital: every six to eight weeks. Everyone in the special care unit, a step down from the intensive care unit, knew Anita and Marilyn, her mother. Anita had suffered birth asphyxia and, as a result, severe neurologic damage including seizures, mental retardation, cerebral palsy, and blindness. At sixteen years of age, Anita was never going to learn to drive a car or go to her high school prom. Because of her lack of mobility, she was bed-bound. Because she was bed-bound, she had muscle wasting and skeletal problems. Anita suffered terrible pain because of her twisted spinal column and her limbs, which were fixed at stiff angles due to muscle contractures. Because she had gastro-esophageal reflux and was unable to clear her oral secretions, she frequently aspirated and had recurrent bouts of pneumonia, the primary reason she was hospitalized so often.

Every time Anita was hospitalized, the physicians tried to discuss DNR orders with her mother. In the event of a cardiopulmonary arrest, the hospital staff was required to resuscitate Anita unless there were specific orders in her chart to the contrary—DNR orders. But Marilyn would not hear of it. Anita was her life. Marilyn was so devoted to her daughter that she willingly undertook the enormous nursing care, including changing adult-size diapers, required for Anita to live at home. In fact, Anita always had perfectly mani-cured fingernails and toenails. Marilyn claimed red was Anita's favorite color, though we couldn't really ask Anita if this was true. She did not speak in words nor use sign language. But her mother always seemed to know if she was happy or angry or in pain.

I didn't know what to make of Anita and Marilyn. Was it possible that although Anita could not communicate with the rest of the world, she could convey her feelings to her mother? Maybe. Who was I to judge?

I dreaded more questions while Baby Boy Smith's mother wept and his father stood stoically without saying a word. I shifted my weight and pulled my white doctor's coat closed, wishing it was armor. Finally, I said I needed to get back to the nursery to take care of their baby. I asked for their consent to send him to Children's Hospital for further treatment; I told them it was in their baby's best interest. I asked if they had any more questions, and they shook their heads.

Just as I stepped out into the hallway, I heard my name. I turned around. The baby's father stood with his hands tunneled into his pockets.

"Doctor, we want you to know his name is Matthew. We'd like everyone to know that."

"Yes, Mr. Smith, I understand."

I tried to put a smile on my face. "Matthew is a nice name."

"We sure do appreciate what you did for our son, Doctor."

He smiled, abashed, face flushed, gratitude in his eyes.

I could not say thank you; I couldn't even look him in the eye. "That's all right, Mr. Smith."

I walked away trying not to think about what I had learned. Baby Boy Smith had parents. Baby Boy Smith had a name.

After the helicopter transport team left with the baby in a flurry of activity, Suzanne immediately set to putting her nursery back in order. The glass room quickly began to bear no signs that a baby once lay there with life-sustaining machinery keeping time in beeps and clangs. I lingered while she wiped away all reminders that something had happened there.

When David came bounding into the nursery to relieve me, Suzanne and I were talking about Halloween costumes for our children. He joined our conversation right away without even asking what we were talking about. David is stocky, of average height, with a head of thick blond hair which seems to be in constant motion, like the rest of his body. David is incapable of being still; he fidgets, taps, shakes incessantly. I gave him a summary of the day's events to the impatient beat of a rubber band snapping in his hand.

"You know he's going to be a vegetable," David blurted out.

I closed my eyes. "Please don't say that."

"You know that, don't you? You are lying to yourself if you don't know that," he gestured impatiently. David talked with his hands.

"Listen, David, I don't want to talk about that right now. I cannot think about what is going to happen to him. I will start crying, okay?" I raised my voice in anger.

"You saved his life. It's not your responsibility to take care of him after this. You did your job," David shrugged.

"*Did I*, David? Did I really help him? Is *he* better off alive and brain-damaged than dead? Are his *parents* better off?" I sat with my head in my hands.

"It's not our job as doctors to question," David dismissed my misgivings.

"Why not? If it's not our job as doctors, whose job is it? You know, this wasn't supposed to happen to me. *This* is the reason I didn't become a neonatologist. I could not deal with the moral and ethical dilemmas," I said in frustration.

"Yeah, I know. As a neonatologist, you save a twenty-five-week preemie and you wonder what you saved. Plus you have to justify the cost in the *raging* debate about the allocation of health-care dollars—do you immunize a thousand kids against polio *or* do you spend the money keeping one premature baby alive?" David asked rhetorically.

"Or one neurologically devastated full-term baby," I said sadly.

I did not want to debate the proper allocation of health-care dollars. We could talk about health-care policy and statistics, but in the end, those issues had names and faces: Matthew Smith, Anita Rogers, Joshua Bennet. I could not escape them. I also could not escape the Hippocratic Oath. "First, do no harm."

I left the hospital that night wondering what I had done. In five short minutes which seemed a lifetime, while I waited for a blue baby to take his first breath, I had sealed the fate of a child and his parents. If Dennis Sullivan had been less skilled and taken more time extracting this baby from his mother's womb, he would have been born truly dead. If I had not been able to push the breathing tube past his vocal cords, he would have remained dead. Instead, he lived.

At the time this happened, the law was pretty clear, but the ethical implications of what I had done were not. I could have been brought up on medical misconduct charges, my license revoked and even criminal charges brought against me if I did not heed the call to save a viable full-term baby. And it would have gone against everything in my training as a doctor to stand by and refuse to resuscitate this baby because of my nagging suspicion that he would be severely brain-damaged. But how viable was he?

That is what the medical community has not answered. The American Academy of Pediatrics has no policy statement to guide pediatricians on the viability of full-term infants resuscitated in delivery rooms. The neonatal resuscitation guidelines suggest, rather than mandate, that an infant with no significant response to heroic measures—i.e., intubation, chest compressions, medications—after fifteen minutes should be pronounced dead and resuscitation ceased. But it does not address what a physician should do when a baby has been born dead for twenty minutes. This dilemma falls in the gray area—that strange and shifting zone where things are neither black nor white, neither right nor wrong.

Although many people praised my life-saving skills, I could not escape the feeling that I had violated the Hippocratic Oath. I did harm. I could not excuse myself. Two months later I resigned as Instructor of Pediatrics and faculty member of the Division of General Pediatrics at one of the most prestigious children's hospitals in the country. I left the world of pediatric hospitalist and joined the world of most general pediatricians—well-child visits, ear infections, colds. I did not want to make any more life-and-death decisions.

But I still think about Baby Boy Smith. I wonder if he is at home or in a hospital or a long-term-care institution. I wonder if his parents think about the doctor who saved their son's life and created a lifelong burden.

•

A former assistant professor of pediatrics at Children's Hospital of Pittsburgh, **Helena Studer** *has practiced pediatrics and taught at St. Christopher's Hospital for Children, the Children's Hospital of Philadelphia, and the Johns Hopkins Hospital. She was born in Kwangju, South Korea, and raised in Uganda, East Africa, and the United States. She currently lives in Pittsburgh, Pennsylvania, with her husband and two children.*

About the Editor

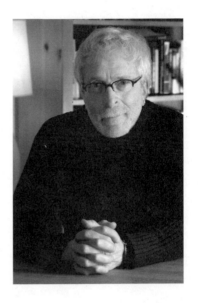

LEE GUTKIND is the founder and editor of *Creative Nonfiction*. He teaches in the Creative Writing Program at the University of Pittsburgh and is a prolific author whose diverse works include *Forever Fat: Essays by the Godfather; The Best Seat in Baseball, but You Have to Stand: The Game as Umpires See It; Many Sleepless Nights: The World of Organ Transplantation;* and *Stuck in Time: The Tragedy of Childhood Mental Illness.* He has edited many collections, including *A View from the Divide: Creative Nonfiction on Health and Science.*

Rage and Reconciliation:
Inspiring a Health Care Revolution

CD Contents

Part I

Introduction, by Lee Gutkind

Excerpts from the essays:

Notes from a Difficult Case, by Ruthann Robson
Read by Helena Ruoti

Burden of Oath, by Linda Peeno, M.D.
Read by Kathryn Spitz

Panel Discussion:
Gary Fischer, M.D.
Karen Wolk Feinstein, Ph.D.
Loren Roth, M.D.
Linda Peeno, M.D.

Host: Lee Gutkind
Director: W. Stephen Coleman
Producer: Laura Jackson
Project Coordinator: Brenda L. Smith
Sound Engineer: Brad Peterson

Thanks for support to the Juliet Lea Hillman Simonds Foundation, the Pennsylvania Humanities Council, the Falk Medical Fund, and the Jewish Healthcare Foundation.

Part II

A Measure of Acceptance, by Floyd Skloot
Read by Don Wadsworth

Closing Remarks, by Lee Gutkind

Host: Lee Gutkind
Director: Amy Hartman
Producer: Laura Jackson
House Manager: Jeff Anderson
Sound Engineers: Robert Deaner and Pete
Matarangelo

Thanks for support to the American Library Association, the National Endowment for the Arts, the John S. and James L. Knight Foundation, the DeWitt Wallace-Reader's Digest Fund, the Pennsylvania Humanities Council, and the Carnegie Library of Pittsburgh.